THE MANAGEMENT OF CLINICAL TRIALS

Edited by **Hesham Abdeldayem**

The Management of Clinical Trials
http://dx.doi.org/10.5772/intechopen.70212
Edited by Hesham Abdeldayem

Contributors

Ivonne Schulman, Russell Saltzman, Daniel DaFonseca, Lina Caceres, Cindy Delgado, Marietsy Pujol, Kevin Ramdas, Jairo Tovar, Mayra Vidro-Casiano, Joshua Hare, Wayne Balkan, Donato Bonifazi, Giulia Chiaruttini, Mariagrazia Felisi, Mariangela Lupo, Angelica Intini, Doriana Filannino, Hesham Abdeldayem

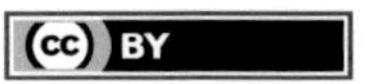

Notice

First published in London, United Kingdom, 2018 by IntechOpen
IntechOpen is the global imprint of INTECHOPEN LIMITED, registered in England and Wales, registration number: 11086078, The Shard, 25th floor, 32 London Bridge Street
London, SE19SG – United Kingdom
Printed in Croatia

British Library Cataloguing-in-Publication Data
A catalogue record for this book is available from the British Library

Additional hard copies can be obtained from orders@intechopen.com

The Management of Clinical Trials, Edited by Hesham Abdeldayem
p. cm.
Print ISBN 978-1-78923-238-7
Online ISBN 978-1-78923-239-4

For EU product safety concerns:
IN TECH d.o.o., Prolaz Marije Krucifikse Kozulić 3, 51000 Rijeka, Croatia, info@intechopen.com or visit our website at intechopen.com.

Meet the editor

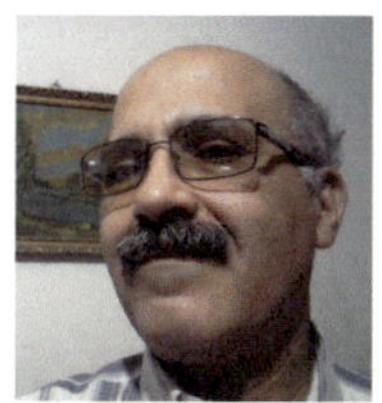

Professor Abdeldayem graduated from Kasr Al-Ainy Faculty of Medicine, in 1987. He got his training at Cairo University Hospitals, National Liver Institute, Ysbyty Gwynedd, Bronglais General Hospital, General Hospital Ayr, University of Pittsburgh Medical Center, and King Abdulaziz Medical City. He joined the National Liver Institute in 1993. He has several publications in the fields of hepato-pancreato-biliary surgery and organ transplantation. He currently holds the positions of Professor of Surgery and the dean at the National Liver Institute, Menoufia University, Egypt.

Contents

Section 1

Introduction

Chapter 1

Introductory Chapter: Introduction to Clinical Trials

Hesham Abdeldayem

Additional information is available at the end of the chapter

http://dx.doi.org/10.5772/intechopen.77285

1. Clinical research

Clinical research may be defined as the research in which an investigator directly deals with human subjects or on material of human origin. It includes mechanisms of human disease, therapeutic interventions, development of new technologies, epidemiologic and behavioral studies, and outcomes and health services research. Types of clinical research may be classified as **retrospective/prospective** that refers to the time of data collection. In prospective studies, the data are collected after the objectives are set. On the other hand, in retrospective studies, the data are collected before the objectives are set. Another classification is **cohort/ cross-sectional studies**. In cohort studies, the subjects are followed over time. On the other hand, in cross-sectional study, the subjects are examined at one point of time, e.g., prevalence of a disease [1].

1.1. Types of clinical research

1. **Case reports**
2. **Observational studies**: Data are collected for a set of patients without randomization.
3. **Clinical trial**: A prospective study evaluating the effect and value of intervention(s) in human subjects under pre-specified settings.

Clinical trials are considered the heart of all medical advances and the "Gold Standard" of clinical research. They are the most definitive tool for evaluation of the applicability of clinical research with the potential to improve the quality of health care and control costs. In other words, they bridge the gap between basic science and improved human health, as they investigate new ways to prevent, detect, or treat diseases or to improve the quality of life [2].

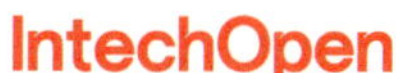

Single center/multi-center trials: Multicenter trials enhance generalizability of the results. In multicenter studies, the use of a central lab makes data handling easier because there is only one set of reference ranges.

2. Non-comparative/comparative design

Noncomparative design is usually used to assess a treatment's safety and tolerability and also in some therapeutic confirmatory studies if long-term safety data are required.

Comparative design is used when comparing treatments: controlled clinical trials groups are studied and contrasts made between groups. Different types of controls include: Historical/ Concurrent: Concurrent controls include placebo and active control (standard therapy or use another new therapy) or "sham" treatment control, e.g., sham surgery or acupuncture. The two most commonly used designs are [3]:

1. **Cross-over**: Each subject receives one treatment and then (after a wash out period) crosses over to receive the other treatment. The individual subject variability is minimized, hence the need for less number of subjects. This design should include an adequate wash out period to ensure baseline status before giving the second treatment, the diseases in question must be stable; otherwise, it will not be considered ethical.
2. **Parallel-group**: Each subject receives only one of the study treatments for a predetermined period, individual subject variability must be taken into account, hence the need for a larger number of subjects [4].

2.1. Selection criteria: Inclusion and exclusion criteria

Selection criteria define which subjects to include and which to exclude. The intension is to identify the appropriate participants in a tightly defined population, based on factors as age, gender, the type and stage of the disease, previous treatment history, and other medical conditions. Examples of exclusion criteria include concomitant therapy that may affect the course of the disease or may lead to drug interactions, women of child bearing potential, pregnant women, nursing mothers, and subjects who cannot comply with protocol (alcoholics or drug users).

3. Research bias

Selection/allocation bias occurs when researcher knows which with the possibility of being tempted to give the treatment under investigation either to subjects who had failed on previous therapy or to those who they think will do well. To eliminate selection bias, studies are conducted on a randomized fashion.

Observer bias is when the investigator knows which treatment a study subject is taking with the possibility that subjects taking a new treatment may be over-scored. To eliminate observer bias, studies are conducted blind [5].

4. Randomization and blinding

Randomization: A process based on allocation of subjects to treatment groups by chance, aiming at removing the potential bias in treatment assignment whether conscious or subconscious. This will greatly enhance the validity of the trial.

Blinding is when the investigator and/or the study subject do not know which subject is taking which treatment. The investigator, the participant, and sometimes even the evaluator are all kept unaware (blinded) of the outcomes of the trial.

1. Single-blinded study: either the investigator or the subject tested is blinded to the intervention allocation.
2. Double-blinded study: both the investigator and the subject tested are unaware about of the intervention allocation.
3. Triple-blinded study: even the evaluator is also not aware of the process.

In emergencies and life threatening situations for participants, unblinding can be done.

Standard operating procedures (SOPs) ensure that the specific tasks in the trial are carried out in a consistent manner. Topics for SOPs for investigators:

1. Ethics: initial and continuing review by ethics committees, informed consent, consent forms, and information sheets
2. Study setup: review of investigator brochures, protocols, protocol amendments, CRFs, and agreements (e.g., responsibility, financial, confidential, and insurance/indemnity agreement)

5. Basic documents and materials of clinical trials

5.1. Protocol

The protocol is a written agreement between investigators, participants, and the scientific community. The protocol must inform (study staff) about how the study treatments will be assigned, how the subjects are to be treated, and what assessments are to be performed. It is the reference comprehensive operational manual that describes **who** is conducting the trial, **who** is sponsoring it, **where** is it to be conducted, and **on whom** it will be conducted, **what** is being tested?, **why** is this research needed, **what** are the risks?, **what** are the procedures?,

how will data be collected, **how many** patients you will need?, and **what** is to be done in any eventuality? It specifies the standard operation procedure (SOP). It describes the background, objective(s), design, methodology, statistical considerations, and organization of the trial. It represents a guideline for the conduct, quality control of a clinical trial, and guidelines to the monitoring groups. It is considered as a legal document for regulatory bodies and may be used to procure funding. It should contain the right amount of detail necessary for the reader of each section to be able to understand exactly what is required to conduct the study [5].

6. Specific objectives

6.1. Primary objective

It defines one question the investigators are most interested in answering and is capable of being adequately answered. It should define the **primary endpoint,** which is a defined measurement or assessment. If possible, end-points need to be objective measurements rather than subjective outcomes. However, many diseases necessitate measurements of subjective symptoms, e.g., pain, discomfort, irritation, etc. Ideally, a clinical trial has just one end point, and this is the primary end point. Common failing is too many end points. The best designed trials keep it simple as this makes a clear answer more likely and easier to achieve.

6.2. Secondary objectives

Secondary objectives should be based on subgroup hypotheses that are respectively defined and based on reasonable expectations and should not distract from the primary objective.

Methods include hypothesis, patient population, inclusion criteria, exclusion criteria, and trial design.

Protocol amendment: A written description of a change(s) to or formal clarification of a protocol. Must be approved by IRB prior to implementation may be partial or complete.

7. Phases of clinical trials

Phase 0: Preclinical animal studies.

Phase I: First-time test of intervention in a small group of people (20–80) to evaluate safety, determine appropriate dosage, and identify side effects. Follows successful pharmacological and toxicological studies in animals start with 1/5th or 1/10th maximum tolerated dose in the most sensitive animal species.

Phase II: Intervention given to a larger group (100–300) to evaluate effectiveness and safety. First administered to patients. Phase IIa (early phase II) potential benefits and side effects establish dose range for phase IIb. Phase IIb (late phase II) establishes efficacy in specific disease. Compare efficacy and side effects with other drugs for same conditions.

Phase III: Randomized, controlled, double-blinded. A sufficient sample size for statistical evaluation of efficacy and safety. Intervention given to large groups (1000–3000) to confirm effectiveness, monitor side effects, compare to other treatments, and collect information that will allow it to be used safely. Successful phase III trial leads to request permission to market new drug.

Phase IV: After drug obtained marketing license, post marketing studies determine additional information including risks, benefits, and optimal use of an intervention [6].

8. Ethical considerations

Every possible precaution should be taken to ensure the safety of research participants including uncoerced and truly informed consent ensuring that the research staff conducts the study honestly and thoroughly.

8.1. Evolution of research ethics guidelines

1. Nuremburg "Doctor's Trial": 1946 in response to Nazi atrocities of using concentration camp prisoners for human experiments.
2. Nuremburg: 1947
3. UN Universal Declaration of Human Rights: 1948
4. Declaration of Helsinki: 1964
5. Belmont Report: 1979
6. International Ethical Guidelines for Biomedical Research (CIOMS): 1993 (Updated 2002)

The Declaration of Helsinki: A set of principles defining the standards that should apply to biomedical research worldwide. It remains the cornerstone ethical reference for global medical research. It is a statement of clinical principles to provide guidance to physicians and other participants in medical research involving human participants.

Informed consent: It is a process by which the participant voluntarily confirms the willingness to participate in a particular clinical research trial, after having been informed of all aspects of the trial that are relevant to the subject's decision to participate. It consists of two parts: a written information describing the clinical trial and a form which the subject signs to document that he/she has given consent to take part in the study and obtained from the participants in the study population after explaining them fully about the purpose, duration, required procedures, expectations, risks and benefits, adverse effects of the trial if any, participants' rights and compensation and/or treatment available to subject in the event of trial-related injury. It is a process not just signing a form communication document not having a legal binding on the patients. The consent should state that the subject's participation is voluntary and that he/she may refuse to participate or withdraw from the trial at any time [5, 7].

Author details

Hesham Abdeldayem

Address all correspondence to: habdeldayem64@hotmail.com

National Liver Institute, Menoufia University, Egypt

References

[1] Francis D, Roberts I, Elbourne DR, Shakur H, Knight RC, Garcia J, Snowdon C, Entwistle VA, McDonald AM, Grant AM, Campbell MK. Marketing and clinical trials: A case study. Trials. 2007;**8**:37. DOI: 10.1186/1745-6215-8-37

[2] Medical Research Council. Clinical Trials for Tomorrow. London: MRC; 2003

[3] Prescott RJ, Counsell CE, Gillespie WJ, Grant AM, Russell IT, Kiauka S, Colthart IR, Ross S, Shepherd SM, Russell D. Factors that limit the quality, number and progress of randomised controlled trials. Health Technology Assessment. 1999;**3**(20):1-143

[4] Bammer G. Enhancing research collaborations: Three key management challenges. Research Policy. 2008;**37**:875-887. DOI: 10.1016/j.respol.2008.03.004

[5] Edwards P. Questionnaires in clinical trials: Guidelines for optimal design and administration. Trials. 2010;**11**:2. DOI: 10.1186/1745-6215-11-2

[6] Schulz KF, Altman DG, Moher D. The CONSORT group: CONSORT 2010 statement: Updated guidelines for reporting parallel group randomised trials. BMJ. 2010;**340**:c332. DOI: 10.1136/bmj.c332

[7] Moher D, Hopewell S, Schulz KF, Montori V, Gøtzsche PC, Devereaux PJ, Elbourne D, Egger M, Altman DG. The CONSORT group: CONSORT 2010 explanation and elaboration: Updated guidelines for reporting parallel group randomised trials. BMJ. 2010:340. DOI: c869-10.1136/bmj.c869

Section 2

Paediatric Clinical Trials

Chapter 2

Challenges in Paediatric Clinical Trials: How to Make It Feasible

Giulia Chiaruttini, Mariagrazia Felisi and
Donato Bonifazi

Additional information is available at the end of the chapter

http://dx.doi.org/10.5772/intechopen.72950

Abstract

The number of paediatric clinical trials in EU has remarkably increased in the last decade in response to the implementation of the new Paediatric Regulation and incentives aiming to define the need of child-specific drug development. Nevertheless, the gap between the number of paediatric and adult-randomised controlled trials is still substantial in almost every major clinical specialty. Economic, ethical, technological, geographical and cultural factors can influence the paediatric drug development and can represent the challenges to be faced for a smooth conduction of a paediatric clinical trial. The need for trials and paediatric patient's engagement to commensurate with the approved paediatric investigation plans is so high that it is crucial to correctly address key factors. Particular care should be taken to develop well-designed studies, with efficient management plans, experienced administrative and healthcare personnel, awareness of socio-cultural features of the geographic areas involved and good communication with patients and their families in order to ensure 'trial preparedness'. A case study on a multinational paediatric clinical trial, presented within the recently ended research project 'DEferiprone Evaluation in Paediatrics (DEEP)', was reported to exemplify some of the challenges encountered by the authors and the actions taken to overcome them.

Keywords: paediatric clinical trial, children medicines development, clinical trial management, ethics, patient enrolment, trial preparedness, drug formulation, regulatory, patient engagement

1. Introduction

Paediatric clinical research was introduced in response to the increasing gaining of awareness that paediatric subjects cannot simplistically be defined as 'small-scale' adults but that possess

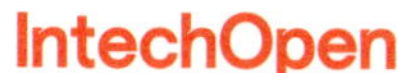

a unique and constantly evolving set of physiological, mental and metabolic characteristics that require a dedicated exploration to identify their appropriate needs.

Before the introduction of international regulations and incentives aiming to define the need of child-specific drug development, paediatric subjects were systematically given off-label treatments, which did not possess any efficacy or safety data for their specific population but that were only tested in adults. The reason for this lack of interest lies on a lower market appeal, together with the fact that the design and execution of clinical trials in children have always been on one hand a controversial matter, with very delicate ethical implications to be considered and consequently regulated, and on the other hand a difficult process, with low number of patients, intrinsically fragmented in further subgroups and with a need of tailored formulations.

2. Historical perspectives

The milestone that signed the beginning of the modern paediatric clinical research, with care in defining the proper requirements and ethical issues related to this vulnerable population, was represented by the introduction of the first international regulations on paediatric subjects.

These regulations have been defined independently in the most developed countries, but in accordance to unified guidelines suggested by the ICH, an organization working on the harmonization of pharmaceutical regulatory requirements within the EU, Japan and the USA.

2.1. Definition of paediatric population

Defining the paediatric population is a very complex task, as it encloses a very broad and multifaced spectrum of subjects. The international regulation on paediatric clinical trials [1] has subdivided it in further four subsets: pre-term and term neonates (0–27 days), infants (1–23 months), children (2–11 years) and adolescents (12–18 years). According to the recently revised EMA guideline 'Ethical considerations for clinical trials on medicinal products conducted with minors' issued on September 2017, the age groups of children and adolescents have been further redefined into pre-schoolers (2–5 years), schoolers (6–9 years) and adolescents (10–18 years) [2]. The latter age group is based on the WHO definition of adolescence starting at the age of 10 years but maybe it has to be further subdivided into two subgroups because it seems to the authors to be too wide. Age groups can be differently subdivided, and often these categories are only used to provide guidance for regulatory and clinical reasons but do not reflect the maturity of the individuals, which is something that is generally recognized as crucial aspect to be taken into account during the conduct of paediatric clinical trials. Given these uniqueness, nonetheless, international paediatric regulations try to create a unified system of rules and laws, aiming to define the needs and protect the entire paediatric population.

2.2. European Paediatric Regulation

The European Paediatric Regulation was adopted in 2006 and entered into force in 2007. It 'lays down rules concerning the development of medicinal products for human use in order to meet the specific therapeutic need of the paediatric population, without subjecting the paediatric population to unnecessary clinical or other trials and in compliance with Directive 2001/20/EC' ([3], Article 1).

Since its implementation, the Paediatric Regulation has a very positive impact on paediatric drug development. The 10-year report of the EMA has shown that it has led to more medicines for children, better and more information for prescribers and patients, better paediatric research and development, more regulatory support for paediatric matters and paediatrics now being an integral part of medicine development [4].

Main sections ruled by the Regulation are:

- the institution of the PDCO;
- the definition of the regulatory requirement for a marketing authorization, among which the PIP;
- the introduction of rewards and incentives for the development of paediatric drugs, i.e., the PUMA.

2.2.1. PDCO

The Paediatric Committee is composed of independent and impartial members appointed from Member States, health professionals, and patients' associations. In its whole, the PDCO provides scientific competences on the main areas of the paediatric medicines, such as drug development, paediatric medicine, physics, paediatric pharmacology, pharmacovigilance, ethics and public health. Its main roles are:

- to assess and give a final opinion on the content and compliance of PIPs, waivers and deferrals;
- to give advice on issues related to surveys on the use of medicinal products in paediatric patients, to the establishment of a European network for paediatric research (EnprEMA) and to the elaboration of documents related to the Regulation;
- to establish a specific and updated inventory of paediatric medicinal product needs.

2.2.2. PIP

The Paediatric Investigation Plan is a document that describes timing and measures by which the developer of an IMP proposes the assessment of quality, safety and efficacy of that IMP in all the concerned subsets of paediatric population, giving also indications of the measures to be taken to adapt the formulation of the product to the needs of each paediatric population. It must be drawn up and submitted to the PDCO at the EMA with a request of agreement before any application for marketing authorisation and possibly not later than upon completion of the human pharmacokinetic studies in adults. The PDCO is in charge of the assessment of the PIP and may request further clarifications and modifications to the applicant. The final opinion can be either positive or negative.

The developer will be granted a *waiver*, if:

- the IMP and the proposed plan are judged unsafe or ineffective in some subset or in the whole paediatric population;
- the IMP does not represent a significant therapeutic benefit over other existing treatments for paediatric patients.

2.2.3. PUMA

The Paediatric Use Marketing Authorisation is a marketing authorisation that gives supplementary protection to a medicinal product for human use exclusively developed for its indication/formulation for paediatric use, where this same medicinal product was already authorized and is not covered anymore by a patent. It is granted to IMPs that have successfully completed an agreed PIP and have set a risk management plan for the follow-up of efficacy and safety of the product. It warrants data and market protection for 10 years.

2.3. American Paediatric Regulations

Paediatric clinical research started in the US few years in advance compared to Europe. The most recent legislation ruling this subject is essentially enclosed in two main acts, i.e., the PREA, also known as 'the paediatric rule' of 2003 [5] and the BPCA, 'paediatric exclusivity' of 2002 [6], both amended in the FDAAA of 2007 [7].

2.3.1. PREA

The Paediatric Research Equity Act defines the regulations on the subject of research into paediatric uses for drugs and biological products. The organ assigned to the assessment and supervision of the paediatric drug development is the Secretary of Health and Human Services, which acts in collaboration with a designated internal committee within the FDA with expertise in paediatrics, biopharmacology, statistics, chemistry, legal issues, paediatric ethics, and appropriate expertise on the products under assessment.

They assess and review application on drugs for paediatric use and are entitled to grant approvals or, in well justified cases, deferrals for the performance of the study in paediatric patients, or even waivers for products not suitable for children or in which the performance of the study is proven highly impracticable. The cases in which the disease and the effects of the drug are similar enough in adults and paediatric patients, an opinion can be issued in which paediatric effectiveness will be extrapolated from well-designed studies in adult patients, maybe with the addition of supplementary data obtained in paediatric subjects such as pharmacokinetics studies.

In addition, the PREA highlights the necessity of a transparent public dissemination of paediatric data obtained either from new products or from marketed drugs for use in adults. It is also duty of the secretary to perform periodic surveys and reviews, analyse data and create statistics on paediatric studies in terms of number of assessments, authorizations, waivers and deferrals, paediatric plans and timelines, formulations, labelling changes and recommendations and report them to the Congress. The suggested channel for the public dissemination of data is the FDA website ([7], title IV).

2.3.2. BPCA

The Best Pharmaceutical for Children Act establishes an incentive system for the performance of paediatric studies with the aim of expanding the number of labels, indications and safety and efficacy information in the different paediatric subgroups. In this case, when the secretary judges that information related to the use of a new drug or an already-marketed drug in the paediatric population would be beneficial on public health, it issues a written request to the sponsor, that for completing such study in a defined timeframe and providing the information requested will be granted an extension of 6 months on market exclusivity ([7], title VI). The BPCA can be considered one of the most successful legislative initiatives, which brought a huge increase in the paediatric studies and the subsequent assignment of paediatric labelling.

3. Challenges in paediatric drug development

Paediatric drug development is hampered by many factors that historically have made it a neglected subject in the pharmaceutical industry's scenario. These factors are of different nature and altogether contribute to the challenge that a sponsor has to face in order to perform and complete a PCT. This section describes these main challenging factors, as a practical overview of the crucial aspects to be considered before the initiation of a PCT, in a perspective of "trial preparedness" (also categorized in **Figure 1**).

3.1. Economic burdens

Drug development is a long, extremely expensive process, with low percentages of success, i.e., final market authorization. The last decades have seen an intensification of the economic challenges, with R&D costs constantly increasing and successfully commercialized products regularly decreasing. In the paediatric research, the economic factor represents a big barrier, as the returns promised by the paediatric market are even more disadvantageous compared to the burden that has to be undertaken. Crucial factors that make paediatric investigation economically more challenging and therefore less profitable are as follows:

- small patient population, which is further fractioned in several subgroups and strongly reduces market's size;
- under-developed infrastructures, which undermine a timely and cost-effective performance of PCTs, i.e., properly GCP-trained paediatric investigators, investigation sites, centralized laboratories and contract research organizations with specific expertise in paediatric trials;

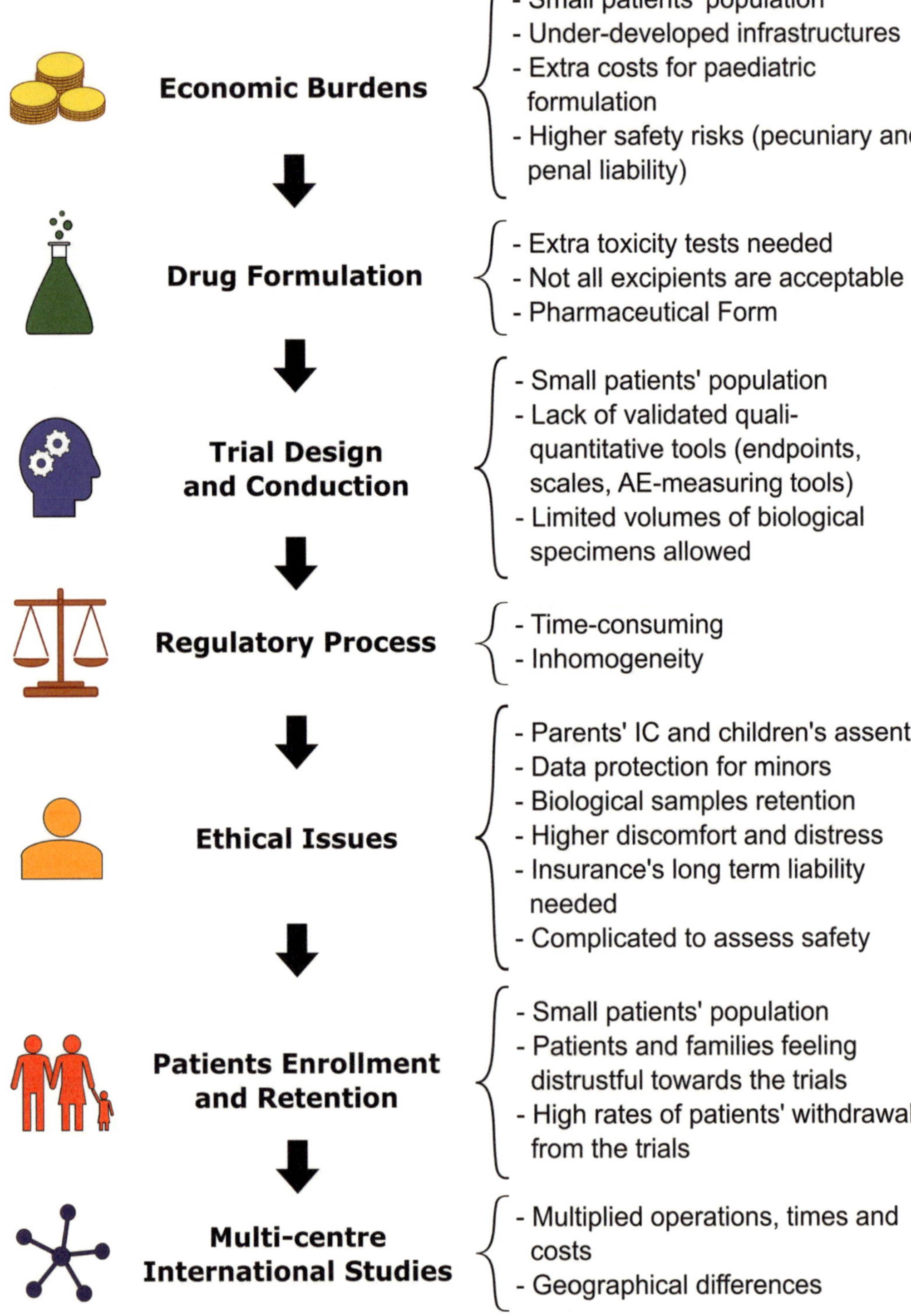

Figure 1. Aspects to consider for trial design. The flowchart summarises the most common drawbacks that can be encountered during the conduct of a paediatric clinical trial.

- need of age-appropriate formulations, that are often very difficult to develop because of the chemical-physical characteristics of the active moieties, the possible adverse reactions of the excipients, the taste, total volume etc. This process is therefore very challenging on a technical point of view, taking long time to complete and making the cost/profit ratio of the drug disadvantageous;
- risks in children can be higher than in adults, with unpredictable serious adverse reactions and long-term effects. These risks may result in pecuniary liability, which represents a strong deterrent for all the parties involved, i.e. sponsors, producers, all levels of healthcare as well as liability insurers.

3.2. Drug formulation

The technological development of a drug for paediatric use is very demanding, and it has to take into consideration many aspects that could be of potential harm for minors or act as a deterrent for a correct and continued administration of the treatment. Therefore, many guidelines have been disseminated by EMA and WHO [8–11] that identify acceptable paediatric drugs' features in terms of quality and formulation.

3.2.1. Drug quality

This aspect is of high importance if we consider the fact that children can be more susceptible to chemicals and bioactive substances, hence it is crucial that the composition of the drug is well known and characterized. ICH provides several guidelines regarding the limits for potentially harmful chemicals to be found in API in the form of impurities, degradation products and solvent residuals [12–15]. These limits apply for both adults and children, with the idea that less quantity will be administered to children. Most of the times, drugs to be used in the younger children's subgroups, i.e., neonates, toddlers, infant and young kids, need further attention, as they require preclinical studies to be performed first on juvenile animals in order to assess possible short- and long-term toxicities, thus increasing the time spent on the final formulation of the drug.

3.2.2. Excipients

According to the working document on paediatric medicines development of the WHO, for the choice of excipients to be used for a paediatric formulation, there should be a consideration on different aspects, e.g., the safety in the target age group, based on the route of administration and the frequency, duration and dosage of treatment [10]. The risks are higher for liquid formulations, but in general, the number of excipients used for a paediatric formulation should be kept to a minimum, as safety data in younger children are mostly limited if not totally missing. Colouring agents and antimicrobial preservatives have quite often toxic and allergenic potential and should be avoided as far as possible, e.g., favouring solid formulations to the liquid ones. This last solution has however negative consequences on the appropriateness of intake by younger children, as they could badly accept them due to the inability to swallow tablets. Sweetening agents are another delicate aspect. On one hand, they are often required in liquid formulations to mask an otherwise unpleasant taste of the drug that could compromise the adequate administration and intake of the treatment. On the other hand, sweeteners' possible side effects should be kept in consideration, i.e., cariogenicity, laxative effects, glycaemic spikes in patients with diabetes, inflammatory reactions in patients with fructose intolerance, etc.

3.2.3. Dosage forms

Strength and dosage forms of paediatric drugs are important aspects to ensure a precise and manageable administration of treatment. Ideal formulation should warrant a ready-to-use shape, ideally adjusted on an age-specific need base, meaning more than one dosage form or more than one strength of a dosage form of the API. A minimal dosing frequency should be attempted, therefore favouring prolonged-release to immediate release formulations.

3.3. Trial design

The phase of planning is the most crucial for the smooth and prompt conduct of a clinical trial. Therefore, it requires a consistent amount of groundwork, logical thinking and awareness of the possible risks and complications. This can be even more true in the case of PCT, where the sensible factors to be considered are usually many more and more difficult to solve than for the clinical trials to be performed in adults.

3.3.1. Innovative trial design

Notwithstanding their little spread in the common use, innovative trial design methods are particularly suitable and powerful for facing issues related to low patients' number and control groups of PCTs. Bayesian design allows the extrapolation of results out of fewer children than in the conventional, fixed-number design, also considering evidences on adults [16]. The randomised withdrawal approach is mostly appropriate for long-term illnesses. More innovative trial design methods are being developed, thanks to the use of simulation studies. These methods, thanks to their features, represent a reliable way of ultimately improving paediatric care, by sensibly limiting the number of children required for achieving good-quality and ethical research [17].

3.3.2. The patient's perspective

It is crucial for clinical trial success to design a study with deep consideration of the patients' needs and perspective, such the possible pain or discomfort caused by certain invasive procedures or by interventions during a particularly difficult status of the patient, the length of assessments and interviews, the number of visits, the duration of the study and the frequency of drug intake. Not least, consideration should be given to the delicate aspect of data protection within the category of vulnerable subjects, which minors belong to.

3.3.3. Quali-quantitative assessments

Another obstacle that requires lots of problem-solving capacity in the design of a PCT is the lack of tools and/or methods for quantitative and qualitative assessment tailored for the paediatric population and its subgroups. Examples in which these deficiencies can be found are as follows:

- study endpoints;
- questionnaires and scales for the measurement of psychophysical parameters;
- tools for the assessment of adverse reactions.

The use of scales and tools validated for the analysed patients' age is crucial to guarantee the proper collection and value of data for a trial. Lack of these means can imply the impossibility to proceed with a certain endpoint, thus invalidating the study.

3.3.4. Biological specimens

Many trials require the collection of patient's biological samples for the acquisition of crucial data. The aspect of the blood withdrawal in particular has to be carefully evaluated. On an ethical point of view, there is the need of avoiding as much as possible any kind of discomfort or pain to the child. On a clinical point of view, there is a very limited volume of blood (and other biological samples) that can be drawn from a child [18]. A document of recommendations, produced in 2008 and recently revised by the ad hoc group for the development of implementing guidelines for Directive 2001/20/EC, states that trial-related blood loss should exceed neither 3% total blood volume during a period of 4 weeks nor 1% at any single time [2]. These considerations have to be carefully implemented during trial design, as it can be a reason for rejection by the ethics committee evaluating study regulatory submission.

3.4. Regulatory process

The procedures and times for regulatory approvals in different countries and investigation sites can be very inhomogeneous and time-consuming. Each regulatory body requires a separate process of revision, with comments to be addressed separately. This process is a big drawback in the case of multi-centre international studies, because it could generate different versions of the study protocol that will have to go through a further step of amendment in order to be harmonized among the investigation sites. In the European context, the new Regulation on Clinical Trials foresees the implementation of a centralized system of submissions to speed up and harmonize the process of regulatory approval of clinical studies within EU [19]. When active, this system will allow a single, fully electronic submission through the EU portal for all the Member States concerned. Technical and scientific aspects of the trial application will be discussed jointly, whereas ethical aspects will be appraised separately by the concerned Member States. They will give back opinions and requests of clarification following unified deadlines. Each Member State will then give an individual response to the sponsor through the EMA portal. In conclusion, the centralized submission will be followed by separate authorizations. Studies' information will be then accessible through a unified European database. In preparation to the implementation of this new system, a sort of test version has been introduced in the last few years by the EMA with the VHP, which already allows a much smoother process for study approval in European investigation sites. Nonetheless, the system still needs to be followed by submissions in single countries, and country-specific requirements are still present.

3.5. Ethical issues

Paediatric clinical research has multiple ethical implications that represent a big component in the difficult process of performing paediatric clinical trials.

These implications are the centre of all the regulations that have been implemented on this matter, and still some grey areas persist and are under constant improvement and implementation. Nevertheless, ethical principles have been expressed in lots of documents produced by the most influential organizations worldwide, such as WHO, ICH and EMA [2, 20–23]. Major points are that children should not be subjects of clinical trials when the research can be performed in less vulnerable populations, and if the research is necessary, care should be taken to include first the least vulnerable subgroups. Unnecessary replication of trials in children is considered unethical too.

More generally, PCTs should be conducted following the so-called 'Belmont principles', which are *beneficence* (do good and avoid harm), *justice* (fair distribution of burden and benefits of research) and *respect* to persons [24], and the four healthcare ethics' principles of *autonomy* (rights of patients to take decisions about their medical treatment), *beneficence and non-maleficence* (called just beneficence in the Belmont principle) and *justice* [25].

3.5.1. Informed consent and assent for paediatric groups

The issue of the informed consent in PCTs is very delicate because, on a legal perspective, children cannot provide a consent for themselves. For patients under legal age, informed consent has to be given by the parent(s) or a legal representative. According to the several common guidelines valid within the EU [2, 26], informed consent must be given before patient's enrolment in the trial, and after receiving an adequate information on the purpose of the research, potential risks and benefits related to the involvement of children in the clinical trial, randomization, volunteering nature of the enrolment and absolute freedom to withdraw anytime with no consequences. This information must be provided by experienced investigators, putting no pressure whatsoever and allowing enough time for the parents/legal representative to reflect on it and ask for further information if needed. Communication must be very clear, and the comprehension of the information must be ensured even with the assistance of a mediator if necessary. Informative material must be therefore very clear, complete and easy to read, which is very much valued by ethics committees appraising PCT applications. Children able to a certain degree of understanding of the research should be, as an important principle of ethical research, involved in the process of making decisions about the enrolment in a trial. This involvement must take into consideration the maturity level of the child, so the communication and the informative material prepared must be age appropriate (this aspect is another very important step in the ethics committee evaluation process). The information can be followed by the obtainment of an assent from the child. In general, both consent and assent must be checked by the investigator as part of the normal communication with parents and children for the entire period of the trial. Informed consent must be sought again as soon as possible where a paediatric patient is no longer a minor.

However, despite internationally accepted ethical principles and the EU guidelines, special provisions for children vary between and, in some cases, within countries due to differences in national laws and practices. A unique definition of legal age of consent is lacking, and the validity of assent and age-grouping is therefore not harmonized across Europe. As the EnprEMA marked in the paper 'Informed consent for paediatric clinical trials in Europe', usually the legal age for the informed consent is 18 years, but it differs in some countries: in Austria, it is 14; in Finland and Denmark, it is 15; and in the UK, it is 16 [27]. Specific characteristics in terms of informative material to be provided as well as requirements on the matter of rights of the patient to sign informed consent or assent, whether in addition or not to the parent's consent are detected [27, 28]. Solving this issue is of primary importance in the perspective of implementing the new European Regulation, since the lack of EC practice harmonization will impede the achievement of a unified evaluation of PCT applications at central level.

3.5.2. Data protection and biological samples retention

The major concern about data protection in children regards their possible uses in the future, after the termination of a trial. In this matter personal information are included, in particular regarding sexuality or illicit substance abuse, but also biological samples collected and stored long-term. There is the need of a careful protection of these data. Retention of any material must be consented (and reconsented once the child comes of age) and confidentiality guaranteed.

3.5.3. Discomfort and distress in trial procedures

Given the vulnerable nature of paediatric patients, extra attention must be paid to the discomfort or pain caused to children by trial-related procedures. This is a very important ethical issue that has to be widely considered when designing a PCT, to take all the measures to avoid unnecessary distress in every feasible way. In any case, signs of discomfort, pain and distress must be always measured through the use of validated age-appropriate scales. Appropriate analgesia should be provided where a certain degree of pain is caused by strictly necessary procedures.

3.5.4. Insurance

Insurance is compulsory in order to safeguard patients. In the case of PCTs, it is important to make sure that insurance includes long-term liability. Since this risk is much higher in children than in clinical trials performed in adults, insurance companies are reluctant to provide this protection. Finding the right company can be therefore quite a challenging process in the start-up of a PCT.

3.5.5. Safety

As in every clinical trial, safety must be constantly evaluated and monitored, and adverse events should be always timely reported. Safety in paediatric subjects, given their vulnerability, is very important, but detecting these events can be particularly complicated. First, because children could show effects never seen before in adults, with the consequence of unpredictable manifestations. Second, because especially in neonates and toddlers, the reaction could not be easily detectable, and they do not have the possibility to communicate their symptoms. Third, because some methods for detection of adverse reactions are not validated in children, making this assessment hard and imprecise. Consequence of this issue can be on one hand the missed detection of an adverse reaction or on the other hand (more common) the over-interpretation of symptoms as adverse events and the subsequent withdrawal of patients from studies, contributing to issue of patients' retention.

3.6. Patients enrolment and retention

The problem of low percentages in patients' enrolment and retention in PCTs is an issue that contributes to the failure in reaching the numbers for proper study's completion [29] and therefore has probably the biggest impact on the way a PCT is designed. There is a paucity of eligible paediatric subjects for the majority of studies that is dependent on epidemiologic reasons but also on a high degree of patients withdrawing from the studies as well as patients' families being wary about clinical trial's possible risks. This shortage of patients has to be compensated in most of the cases with the involvement of multiple investigation sites. This choice though is often a double-edged weapon, because on one hand, it improves the chances to reach the minimum number of patients necessary to successfully complete a study, and on the other hand, it substantially extends the time, work and costs required for the obtainment of regulatory approvals to conduct the studies in different sites and/or countries and for the study conduct.

3.6.1. Communication with patients and families

Many reasons can be identified for the scarce rate of patient's recruitment and retention in PCTs, among which the wrong approach or miscommunication with patients and their families. The wrong communication between the clinical staff and patients can be tremendously detrimental, because it can lead to the participant (or potential participant) and his family not understanding correctly the conditions of the study, its aims, benefits and potential risks. They could feel distrustful if the entire process is not explained in a transparent way, or even threatened, if they don't understand correctly the important concept of voluntary participation.

In 2012, following a large consultation phase, the PDCO issued a Concept Paper on the involvement of children and young people in its activities, with the children's best interests as primary consideration [30]. The setup of a child-friendly approach implies a collaborative and continuous action involving paediatricians and healthcare professionals, psychologists, families, and patients. Children and parents should be involved not only in the daily clinical practice but also in the whole study development, revision of clinical study protocols and use of drugs. Healthcare professionals should consider children and families' active participation as a fundamental step to reach consensus and compliance to treatments and to increment patient's enrolment and retention. Furthermore, it is necessary to recognize that a standard model of information is not valid for all age groups; therefore, in addition to parents, children, adolescent and mature minors should receive information in a clear and understandable way for their level of comprehension and maturity. These concepts are clearly underlined also in

http://dx.doi.org/10.5772/intechopen.72950

the consultation document 'Ethical considerations for clinical trials on medicinal products conducted with minors', recently updated to be in line with the new Clinical Trials Regulation 536/2014 [2].

3.6.2. Patients' withdrawal

Many factors that could cause discomfort or be uneasy to be pursued by patients or their families have been related to patient's withdrawal. Most common reasons for withdrawing a paediatric study are the wrong formulation of the drug, i.e., the taste (too bitter or with a taste that does not match the preferences of the population the drug is used on), the pharmaceutical form (tablets, capsules, difficult to swallow for some patient's subgroups or injectable solutions that require assistance and could preclude a normal life for the patient) and the strength (not easily scalable for smaller children). Too many doses of treatment per day can cause withdrawal as well or increase the risk of lack of adherence to the study protocol. Too many hospital visits plus the lack of any form of compensation for the expenses can represent a strong deterrent for parents that have to give up on work days. Distressful procedures such as frequent blood withdrawals should be avoided as well.

3.7. Multicentre international studies

As discussed in Section 2.6, the need to increase the number of paediatric patients enrolled in a study in order to reach an adequate statistical sample, is usually managed with the design of multi-centre studies, often performed in different countries as well. This type of trials has in its turn other problematic consequences.

3.7.1. Time and costs

Performing a trial in multiple locations means that the work will be multiplied. There is the need to localize and make agreements with many structures that comply with all the requirements of the study. The study must be approved by multiple competent authorities and ethics committees that can ask for different clarifications, and this can lead to different versions of the study protocol. Submission packages for these requests of authorization must be tailored from country to country, documents for patients such as informative documents, consent and assent forms, but also labels and protocol synopsis have to be translated in the local languages. Substantial differences in the version of study protocol and documents, consequence of the discussion with the different local CAs and ECs, will probably lead to the necessity of an amendment that implements in one version all the edits and makes a right compromise with all the requirements to be submitted again to all the regulatory bodies for approval. If in some cases, a compromise is not possible because of unconcealable ethical principles, different versions have to be handled provided that the aims and GCP compliance of the study are not affected.

3.7.2. Geographic differences

The conduct of the study could be also affected by geographic issues from country to country, especially in locations outside the EU.

Cultural and social differences will cause a very different process of review of the clinical trial application by the ECs that will point out different ethical aspects also depending on the common sense in their society, filtered by cultural, religious and/or political biases. IMP's formulations could be inappropriate for certain populations, as regards taste, pharmaceutical form and/or storing conditions. Border policies could hinder the proper exchange of biological material, IMP, as well as study-specific equipment. Finding the right compromise with all the different countries' requirements and needs in order to keep a well-coordinated study planning and conduct could be therefore very demanding.

4. Overcoming different issues: a case study on a multicentre multinational PCT

As discussed in the previous section, the performance of a PCT is fulfilled with many obstacles that can compromise its success and final outcome. Good strategy, problem solving and a wide preliminary research and awareness of the issues that could present can improve the chances to successfully complete the study. In this section, we propose some solutions for the issues described above, and we use as example the case study of a recently performed research project, the DEEP. DEEP is a 6-year European Project (FP7) coordinated by Consorzio per Valutazioni Biologiche e Farmacologiche (CVBF), a non-profit research consortium based in Italy, comprising 23 recruiting centres in European and non-European countries, scientific partners from several European countries and a pharmaceutical group based in Canada. The DEEP Project has the specific aim to produce a new oral liquid formulation of deferiprone suitable for paediatric use and to integrate the existing information on deferiprone use in iron-overloaded paediatric patients. It consisted of three studies, DEEP-1, DEEP-2 and DEEP-3 in accordance with the PIP submitted to the EMA-PDCO in February 2011 and amended and finally approved in November 2011. It is to be mentioned that the PIP has undergone several modifications upon PDCO request: the age of patients to be recruited, which was extended including all the paediatric ages (from 1 month to 17 years instead of the previously proposed 2–10 years), the sample size (from 240 patients to 310) and also the comparator (from deferoxamine to the more expensive deferasirox), with a huge increase of time and cost.

The DEEP-1 was a multi-centre, oral single dose experimental and modelling study to evaluate the pharmacokinetics of deferiprone in patients under 6 years of age affected by transfusion-dependent haemoglobinopathies (NCT01740713, *clinicaltrials.gov)*. It was concluded in 2014, providing scientific evidence that the dosage per kilogram of deferiprone used in adults and older children can provide sufficient exposure to ensure efficacy also in younger children. These results allowed children aged under 6 years to start to be recruited in DEEP-2 Safety/Efficacy Study.

The DEEP-2 was a phase III multicentre, randomised, open label, non-inferiority active-controlled trial aiming at comparing the efficacy, in terms of changes of serum ferritin levels and cardiac iron overload, of deferiprone versus deferasirox in paediatric patients affected by hereditary haemoglobinopathies, requiring chronic transfusions and chelation (NCT01825512, *clinicaltrials.gov*). It has involved 393 randomized patients with the FPFV in January 2015 and

http://dx.doi.org/10.5772/intechopen.72950

LPLV in September 2017. The DEEP-3 was a long-term observational safety study which evaluated the nature and incidence of adverse effects of deferiprone in children and adolescents with beta-thalassaemia major. Started in 2013, and ended in October 2015, with 297 patients enrolled in the study, it confirmed that the safety profile of deferiprone in children and adolescents is in accordance with the available data in adults.

4.1. Regulatory

The process for granting regulatory authorization in a multicentre multinational PCT is a big time-consuming factor. Every step (submission of PIP, study approval from CAs of every country and from ECs that can be country-specific or even local for the single centres as it is in Italy) can require several months to be completed. In addition, the legal approach is different among countries: each of them has its own rules governing the submission of CTs. On average, a large part of the regulatory bodies involved in the approval process asks for clarifications and/or changes regarding the study protocol, informative material, etc. In the case of DEEP-2, several issues raised on this topic.

In Tunisia, where trials on non-marketed drugs were not allowed on minors, a special authorisation from the Ministry of Health had to be granted before ECs could approve the study. In Albania, a national Law on clinical trials was absent until July 2014; therefore, it was much harder to obtain regulatory approval there. In Egypt, despite several requests, biological samples' exportation for the centralized analyses was never authorized. In Cyprus, the eligibility of patients under 2 years of age was denied, notwithstanding the European regulation, since the study had already been approved in other European countries. For all these obstacles, it was crucial to have a dedicated regulatory team and to have appointed an external expert Ethics Board that could rapidly deal with all the actions required and solve correlated issues.

4.1.1. Ethics and safety

Since ethical and safety issues are among the major concerns in PCTs, in order to ensure a good quality conduct of the study, with focus on the safety and wellbeing of the paediatric patients, a DSMC and an EB were established for DEEP-2 study. The DSMC's main responsibility was to ensure safety monitoring of patients and quality of statistical methods, whereas EB revised the essential documents and procedures dealing with ethical aspects such as (but not limited to) documents for the ECs, Consent and Assent Forms, protocols, results and reports from the studies. In particular, it suggested interventions aimed to protect children's well-being both in the European and non-European Countries, and the use of studies results in favour of the affected populations. In addition, the EB worked in collaboration with the DSMC on all aspects of data protection and confidentiality.

4.1.2. Extra-European studies

For studies outside Europe, national legislations in matter of clinical trials are still very different, and cultural and social diversity affects a lot the common sense of ethics. This issue was faced in the DEEP-2 study. Actions taken to ease the management of the trial started from the planning of the study. An initial survey was performed to define the legal framework regulating clinical trials in different countries. SOPs were setup and followed to implement a unique procedure and a unique CTA 'package of documents'. Local CROs were employed that had the proper expertise together with the right awareness of socio-cultural and regulatory peculiarities, as well as linguistic fluency. Majority of integrations were asked by the different ethics committees regarding the content of the informed consents and assents, and one of the most controversial and dependent on country-specific cultural influences was the topic of contraception and pregnancy (informative documents for Egyptian female adolescents could not include information regarding contraception, whereas for Greek patients, the insurance had to cover foetus damages even though contraceptive measures were explicitly mentioned in the informed consent form).

4.2. Patient-oriented perspective

On the base of the ethical principles concerning patient's proper information and engagement [2, 30], age-tailored (<6, 7–11, 12–17) information booklets explaining CTs' aims and procedures and what they are going to experience, and assent forms were prepared in the framework of the DEEP-2 study. They were the result of a collaborative effort between pharmacologists, paediatricians, child psychologists, communicators and illustrators. Their aim was to inform the participant child on the study's objectives and procedures and to obtain his/her assent to participate in the study. They were translated in all the six languages of the clinical sites included in the trial (Albanian, Arabic, English, French, Greek, Italian). Furthermore patients, parents and patients' organisations were involved in creating the protocol information package, actively participating in the revision of documents for the children and contributing in the design of the dissemination strategy.

The educational part of the study towards kids and families is very important for the participation and compliance; another aspect that would be beneficial, and thus it would be worthy to contemplate it in a study, is the communication to patients and families of the trial results. In this regard, in the context of the DEEP-2 study, strong importance will be given to the establishment of an adequate form of communication of the results specifically designed for laypersons, meaning that comprehension can be reached and further transmitted by involved subjects and their families. The main principles of the lay communication will be followed, with the design of a summary that can be understood by an audience from the age of 12 years upwards. A child-friendly version of the lay summary will also be prepared to help younger children in understanding trial results.

4.3. Selection of centres

As discussed above, the choice of investigation centres can have a huge impact on the outcome of a PCT. A careful selection of the centres involved in the DEEP-2 study was aimed to involve centres complying with as many of the following criteria as possible:

- being localized in a geographical area where epidemiology of the disease under study is high, and thus many patients can be approached;

http://dx.doi.org/10.5772/intechopen.72950

- availability of a Principal Investigator that has a relevant experience in GCP and PCTs, and is willing to collaborate with a proactive attitude;
- facilities necessary to perform all the diagnostics and procedures required by the study protocol present within the hospital/clinic;
- social and cultural features of the area in which the centre is located likely to allow a good understanding and acceptance of the study and of its requirements and characteristics.

4.4. Quality assurance

As already extensively discussed, the number of patients in PCT is a very limiting factor. It is therefore very important that solid data are collected as far as possible from every single patient enrolled in a study. To this aim, the implementation of SOPs specifically designed for paediatric studies and compliance to GCP principles during the entire duration of the clinical trial must be ensured. Proper training must be organized for all the staff involved, and constant monitoring of the activities has to be performed. The quality of the data derives also from a harmonized method of analysis. This can be achieved for example by the organized collection and analysis of samples by a centralized laboratory to rule out instrument's deviations and ensure standardized results.

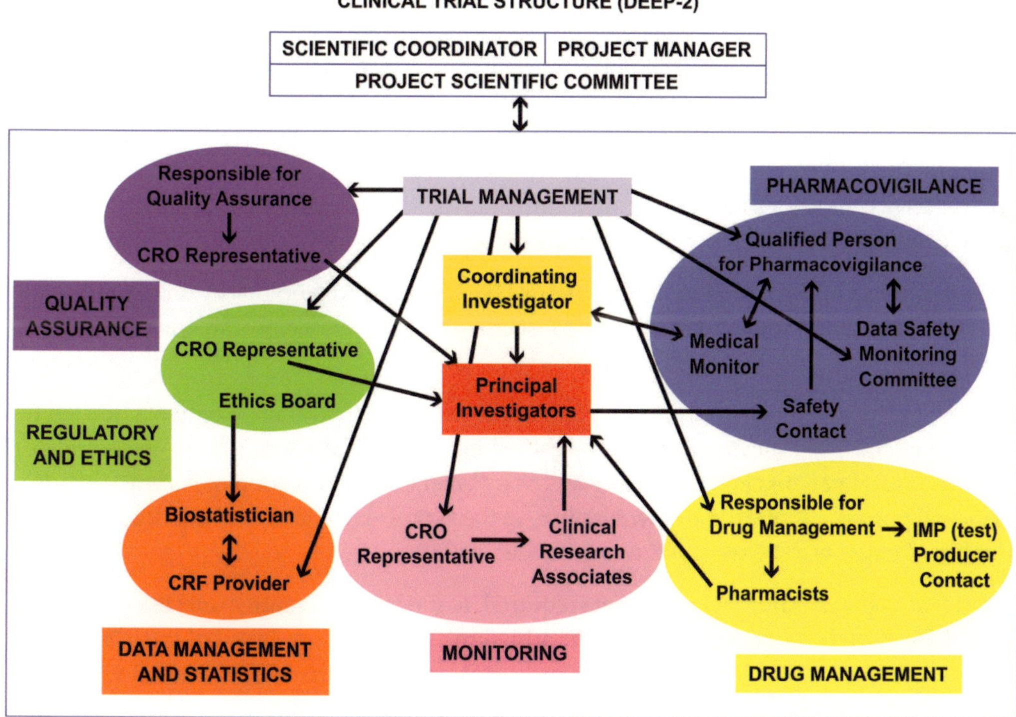

Figure 2. DEEP-2 infrastructure. This schematic depicts the set of organizations and human resources employed for the conduct of DEEP-2 clinical trial in every country it was performed.

This issue was properly addressed in the DEEP-2 study. SOPs were set-up and followed for all the aspects of the trial. A complex trial infrastructure was arranged in order to fulfil all the GCP requirements and promptly respond to all the possible issues and needs arising (**Figure 2**). This infrastructure was made through a well-defined structure of roles and responsibilities for each member of the staff.

Laboratories specialized in pharmacokinetics analysis and blood ferritin diagnostics, were employed for the centralized assessment of these parameters.

In reference to the centralized evaluation of ferritin analysis, a second laboratory was identified within Egypt area due to the impossibility to export biological samples from Egypt which, with its three investigation sites (Alexandria, Cairo and Zagazig), retained almost the 40% of the total samples collected from patients recruited in the entire study. Consistency of data obtained in the two laboratories was ensured using standard controls in both sites for all the analyses performed.

A central laboratory in Australia was assigned for the analysis of images of hepatic R2 and cardiac T2* MRIs acquired and transmitted by the investigation sites. The proper calibration of MRI machines in every centre was ensured with the use of phantoms delivered to the investigation sites.

5. Conclusions

Notwithstanding its important and noble meaning and the possible benefits deriving from its successful conclusion for either society and sponsors, the conduction of PCTs is a path undermined by obstacles and deterrents. We reported the example of DEEP, a European research Project (FP7) coordinated by CVBF and recently concluded. DEEP's final aim was to produce and get the authorization for a new oral liquid formulation of deferiprone with a paediatric indication and to extend the information available on deferiprone in iron-overloaded paediatric patients.

Although successfully completed, many issues had to be faced, and deviations from the initially planned study were the inevitable consequence of the strategies implemented to overcome them.

The first protocol's version reported a population's size of 310 evaluable patients needed for getting statistical significance of data. The estimated drop-out rate was 10%, so the calculated number of total patients to be recruited was 344. When the study started, it became clear that the actual percentage of drop-out was higher, so the protocol had to be amended, and the new number of patients to be recruited was increased to 388.

Because of the higher number of patients required, to the initial 15 centres selected for the conduct of the study, other 8 centres had to be added to allow the recruitment of the 388 patients needed. In actual facts, at the end of the study, 393 patients were randomized, of whom 316 completed the study.

The enrolment rate of patients at different sites was really heterogeneous. In particular, the involvement of two centres respectively in Cairo and Tunis allowed a tremendous number of patients to be recruited because of the high epidemiology of haemoglobinopathies in those countries. On the other hand, in other countries like Greece and Italy, the same successful recruitment rate was not achieved in the same way; possible explanations are a superior diffusion of the prenatal prevention and the presence of more parallel paediatric studies, which have caused a further shrinking of the eligible population.

All the above-mentioned variation to the trial caused an increase in times and costs that were not easily accepted by the European Commission who was funding the initial study program: while a 20 months' project extension was agreed, no additional resources were granted. This caused a tremendous financial stress to all the 16 private and public partners involved in the project (most of them big public hospitals) and only thanks to the contribution from the same partners participating to the project, it was possible to efficaciously conclude it. The anticipated cost of the overall project increased from 7 to 10 million euros.

The study was supposed to be conducted in 3 years, but it took instead 4.5 years in total, plus preliminary activities form PIP submission to study protocol drafting: their duration was supposed to be 1 year long, but it took 3 years instead.

In this chapter, we tried to give the reader a more detailed overview of what obstacles can be encountered during the conduction of a paediatric clinical trial and suggested feasible ways to deal with them, hoping that this under-developed branch of the pharmaceutical research may grow further, providing challenges and opportunities for the next future, and may lead to the successful labelling of new treatments for the paediatric population.

List of abbreviations

API	active pharmaceutical ingredients
BPCA	Best Pharmaceutical for Children Act
CA	Competent authority
CRO	Contract Research Organization
CT	Clinical trial
DEEP	DEferiprone Evaluation in Paediatrics
DSMC	Data Safety Monitoring Committee
EB	Ethics Board
EC	Ethics Committee
EMA	European Medicines Agency
EnprEMA	European network for paediatric research at the European Medicines Agency
EU	European Union

FDAAA	Food and Drug Administration Amendments Act
FPFV	First patient first visit
GCP	Good clinical practice
ICH	International Conference on Harmonisation
IMP	Investigational Medicinal Product
LPLV	Last patient last visit
MRI	Magnetic resonance imaging
PCT	Paediatric Clinical Trial
PDCO	Paediatric Committee
PIP	Paediatric Investigation Plan
PREA	Paediatric Research Equity Act
PUMA	Paediatric Use Marketing Authorisation
SOP	Standard operating procedure
VHP	Voluntary harmonization procedure
WHO	World Health Organization

Author details

Giulia Chiaruttini[1], Mariagrazia Felisi[1,2] and Donato Bonifazi[1,3*]

*Address all correspondence to: ceo@cvbf.net

1 PHARM – Pharmaceutical Research Management SRL, Lodi, Italy

2 CVBF–Consorzio per le Valutazioni Biologiche e Farmacologiche, Pavia, Italy

3 CVBF–Consorzio per le Valutazioni Biologiche e Farmacologiche, Bari, Italy

References

[1] ICH. E11—Clinical Investigation of Medicinal Products in the Paediatric Population. Available at: http://www.ich.org/fileadmin/Public_Web_Site/ICH_Products/Guidelines/Efficacy/E11/Step4/E11_Guideline.pdf [Accessed 19 July 2010]

[2] EudraLex. Ethical Considerations for Clinical Trials on Medicinal Products Conducted with Minors, Revision 1. Available at: https://ec.europa.eu/health/sites/health/files/files/eudralex/vol-10/2017_09_18_ethical_consid_ct_with_minors.pdf [Accessed 17 September 2017]

[3] European Parliament and Council. Regulation (EC) No 1901/2006 of the European Parliament and of the Council. Available at: https://ec.europa.eu/health//sites/health/files/files/eudralex/vol-1/reg_2006_1901/reg_2006_1901_en.pdf [Accessed 12 December 2006]

[4] EMA. 10-year Report to the European Commission—General Report on the Experience Acquired as a Result of the Application of the Paediatric Regulation. Available at: https://ec.europa.eu/health/sites/health/files/files/paediatrics/2016_pc_report_2017/ema_10_year_report_for_consultation.pdf [Accessed 26 October 2016]

[5] 108th US Congress. Pediatric Research Equity Act of 2003. Available at: https://www.congress.gov/108/plaws/publ155/PLAW-108publ155.pdf [Accessed 3 December 2003]

[6] 107th US Congress. Best Pharmaceuticals for Children Act. Available at: https://www.congress.gov/107/crpt/srpt79/CRPT-107srpt79.pdf [Accessed 3 October 2001]

[7] Congress of the United States of America. Food and Drug Administration Amendments Act of 2007. Available at: https://www.fda.gov/downloads/Drugs/DevelopmentApprovalProcess/DevelopmentResources/UCM049870.pdf [Accessed 4 January 2007]

[8] EMA. Reflection Paper: Formulations of Choice for the Paediatric Population. Available at: http://www.ema.europa.eu/docs/en_GB/document_library/Scientific_guideline/2013/07/WC500147002.pdf [Accessed 22 June 2005]

[9] Zajicek A, Fossler MJ, Barrett JS, Worthington JH, Ternik R, Charkoftaki G, Lum S, Breitkreutz J, Baltezor M, Macheras P, et al. A report from the pediatric formulations task force: Perspectives on the state of child-friendly oral dosage forms. The AAPS Journal. 2013;**15**:1072-1081

[10] WHO. Development of paediatric medicines: Points to Consider in pharmaceutical development. Available at: http://www.who.int/medicines/areas/quality_safety/quality_assurance/Rev3-PaediatricMedicinesDevelopment_QAS08-257Rev3_17082011.pdf [Accessed 30 September 2010]

[11] Van Riet-Nales DA, Wang S, Saint-Raymond A, Robert JL. The EMA quality guideline on the pharmaceutical development of medicines for paediatric use. International Journal of Pharmaceutics. 2012;**435**:132-134

[12] ICH. Impurities: Guideline for Residual Solvents Q3C(R6). Available at: http://www.ich.org/fileadmin/Public_Web_Site/ICH_Products/Guidelines/Quality/Q3C/Q3C__R6___Step_4.pdf [Accessed 19 October 2016]

[13] ICH. Guideline for Elemental Impurities Q3D. Available at: http://www.ich.org/fileadmin/Public_Web_Site/ICH_Products/Guidelines/Quality/Q3D/Q3D_Step_4.pdf [Accessed 16 December 2014]

[14] ICH. Impurities in New Drug Products Q3B(R2). Available at: http://www.ich.org/fileadmin/Public_Web_Site/ICH_Products/Guidelines/Quality/Q3B_R2/Step4/Q3B_R2__Guideline.pdf [Accessed 1 June 2006]

[15] ICH. Impurities in New Drug Substances Q3A(R2). Available at: http://www.ich.org/fileadmin/Public_Web_Site/ICH_Products/Guidelines/Quality/Q3A_R2/Step4/Q3A_R2__Guideline.pdf [Accessed 24 October 2006]

[16] Berry DA. Bayesian clinical trials. Nature Reviews Drug Discovery. 2006;**5**:27-36

[17] Baiardi P, Giaquinto C, Girotto S, Manfredi C, Ceci A, TEDDY Network of Excellence. Innovative study design for paediatric clinical trials. European Journal of Clinical Pharmacology. 2011;**67**(Suppl 1):109-115

[18] Howie SR. Blood sample volumes in child health research: Review of safe limits. Bulletin of the World Health Organization. 2011;**89**:46-53

[19] European Parliament. Regulation (EU) No 536/2014 of the European Parliament and of the Council. Available at: https://ec.europa.eu/health//sites/health/files/files/eudralex/vol-1/reg_2014_536/reg_2014_536_en.pdf [Accessed 15 April 2014]

[20] WHO. Declaration of Helsinki. Available at: http://www.who.int/bulletin/archives/79%284%29373.pdf [Accessed 30 September 2001]

[21] UN Documents: Gathering a Body of Global Agreements. Convention on the rights of the child, A/RES/44/25 Annex. Available at: http://www.un-documents.net/crc.htm [Accessed 28 September 2017]

[22] Council of Europe. Convention for the Protection of Human Rights and Dignity of the Human Being with regard to the Application of Biology and Medicine: Convention on Human Rights and Biomedicine. Available at: https://rm.coe.int/168007cf98 [Accessed 3 April 1997]

[23] ICH. Guideline for good clinical practice E6(R1). Available at: https://www.ich.org/fileadmin/Public_Web_Site/ICH_Products/Guidelines/Efficacy/E6/E6_R1_Guideline.pdf [Accessed 9 June 1996]

[24] National Commission for the Protection of Human Subjects of Biomedical and Behavioral Research. The Belmont Report: Ethical Principles and Guidelines for the Protection of Human Subjects of Research. Washington, DC: U.S. Government Printing Office; 1975.

[25] Beauchamp T, Childress J. Principles of Biomedical Ethics. 7th ed. New York: Oxford University Press; 2013

[26] European Commission. Detailed Guidance on the Application Format and Documentation to be Submitted in an Application for an Ethics Committee Opinion on the Clinical Trial on Medicinal Products for Human Use. Available at: https://ec.europa.eu/health/sites/health/files/files/eudralex/vol-10/12_ec_guideline_20060216_en.pdf [Accessed 1 February 2006]

[27] Lepola P, Needham A, Mendum J, Sallabank P, Neubauer D, de Wildt S. Informed consent for paediatric clinical trials in Europe. Archives of Disease in Childhood. 2016;**101**:1017-1025

[28] European Network of Paediatric Research at the EMA. Informed consent for paediatric clinical trials in Europe 2015. Available at: http://www.ema.europa.eu/docs/en_GB/document_library/Other/2015/12/WC500199234.pdf [Accessed 13 June 2017]

[29] Glasser SP. Recruitment and retention in clinical research. In: Glasser SP, editor. Essentials of Clinical Research. Cham: Springer International Publishing; 2014. pp. 177-192

[30] EMA. Concept Paper on the Involvement of Children and Young People at the Paediatric Committee (PDCO). Available at: http://www.ema.europa.eu/docs/en_GB/document_library/Scientific_guideline/2012/09/WC500132555.pdf [Accessed 16 September 2012]

Chapter 3

Informed Participation and Patient Empowerment: A Patient-Centered Approach to Improve Pediatric Clinical Research

Mariangela Lupo, Angelica Intini and
Doriana Filannino

Additional information is available at the end of the chapter

http://dx.doi.org/10.5772/intechopen.74528

Abstract

Over the last years, a Europe-wide trend toward a patient-focused approach is developing and is influencing the decision-making process related to the clinical research. This new vision aims to draw on patient knowledge and experience in order to deliver benefits for all stakeholders of the drug development process, optimizing the clinical study design. In this context, the "patient empowerment" concept has been developed as an approach encouraging the active participation and self-determination of the patients in the caring procedure. For this reason, in 2016, European Patients' Academy (EUPATI) launched a public consultation that ended in September 2016 with the release of the EUPATI guidance for patient involvement in the medicine research and development process. Likewise, the recommendations on the "Summaries of Clinical Trial Results for Laypersons" for the Implementation of Regulation (EU) No 536/2014 recommended a clear and comprehensible communication of the clinical trial results to the patients. However, rarely, all these attempts for the patient involvement pay attention to the pediatric population needs. An innovative approach for the patients' involvement in pediatric clinical research is represented by the **Young Persons Advisory Groups**, an organization composed of youths, patients, and carers, actively participating in clinical research and advising researchers and their teams.

Keywords: patient empowerment, patient involvement, patient-centered approach, child-friendly approach, age-tailored information, patient advocacy, YPAGs—Young Persons Advisory Groups

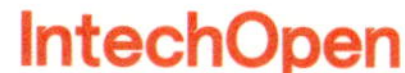

1. Introduction: patient empowerment and involvement

In 1998, the World Health Organization (WHO) released the second edition of the WHO Health Promotion Glossary, where, for the first time, the concept of "Empowerment of the health" was described [1]. **WHO defines empowerment as "a process through which people gain greater control over decisions and actions affecting their health."** In addition, the document makes a difference between community or individual empowerment according to the involvement of individuals acting for themselves or collectively to influence social, economic, and physical conditions impacting their health and quality of life. The WHO Glossary goes on underling that this process, which can be social, cultural, psychological, or political, allows individual or social groups to shed light on what are their needs making clearer what are the efforts required to achieve their goals in life. In this context, the WHO definition also includes a description of health promotion as the process able to create the favorable conditions to convert efforts of individuals and groups into health outcomes as described above [1].

Actually, the concept of empowerment is somewhat complex and includes several psychological and social components that, over the last years, have been studied empirically. In particular, Peter Schulz and Kent Nakamoto underlined the need to distinguish and separate the concepts of empowerment and high health literacy. They are often mismatched, but it is necessary to recognize that they are conceptually and empirically distinct. High literacy, in fact, does not necessarily entail empowerment and vice versa. Furthermore, in order to be sure that the empowerment process is successful, it is important to have both a high literacy and a high degree of mastery. At the same time, the impacts of health literacy and patient empowerment are deeply intertwined, considering that the prevalence of one of them could bring to nonoptimal health outcomes: high levels of health literacy without an adequate degree of patient empowerment can make the patient too dependent on health professionals; while, on the contrary, high degree of empowerment may bring to unsafe health choices if not associated with an appropriate level of health literacy (**Figure 1**).

Finally, the achievement of empowerment by the patient depends on some personal abilities as well as the environmental conditions. In fact, some *life skills* of the patient, such as the scientific approach and the wisdom, are fundamental to acquire the proper knowledge to interact with their healthcare provider. On the other hand, it is essential that the external environment stimulates the patient propensity to be an active protagonist of the healthcare process. The

		Psychological Empowerment	
		Low	High
Health Literacy	High	Needlessly Dependent Patient	Effective Self-manager
	Low	High-needs Patient	Dangerous Self-manager

Figure 1. Relationship between empowerment and health literacy.

healthcare provider should encourage the patients to participate in the care process, avoiding that the patient acts as a passive user.

Overall, four components have been identified as being fundamental to the process of patient empowerment: (1) acquisition by patients of sufficient knowledge to be able to engage with their healthcare provider, (2) patient skills, (3) the presence of a facilitating environment, and (4) understanding by the patient of his/her role.

The transition from empowerment to **patient involvement** implies an important change of attitude: healthcare actors are no longer giving patients their information and allowing them to control the outcomes, but rather they are now actively working to engage patients in their healthcare. In particular, patient participation refers to the involvement of the patient in decision-making or expressing opinions about different treatment methods, which includes sharing information, feelings, and signs, and accepting health team instructions. As a result, the focus has gone from a patient-driven process to a healthcare provider-driven one.

Generally, several studies and European initiatives carried out over the last years have revealed that such patient-centered approach may raise the adequacy of exams and care and reduce the risk of litigation and expenses [2].

2. Patient empowerment: a new frontier in the European scenario

2.1. The European Patients' Academy on therapeutic innovation (EUPATI)

In Europe, the patient-focus approach is becoming a key point in the decision-making process related to the clinical research and an important element of pharma companies' business models and research ethics committees who advocate for the protection of patients in clinical trials. It requires new strategies, new organizational structures, and a culture change across the pharma sector as well as a direct link with patient experts who are capable of providing advice on the value of treatments and on what health outcomes are relevant to patients.

Over the last years, in fact, several initiatives have been carried out with the scope to sensitize the clinical world and encourage the patient involvement in the clinical research. One of the most significant initiatives is the **European Patients' Academy (EUPATI)** [3], funded within "Call 3" of the Innovative Medicines Initiative (IMI) in the period from February 2012 to January 2017, with the scope to prompt a major reflection on the importance of the patient involvement in the medicines development process. EUPATI is a Paneuropean project implemented as a public-private partnership by a collaborative multistakeholder consortium from the pharmaceutical industry, academia, not-for-profit, and patient organizations. Its main activities include the education and training on medicines development, clinical trials, medicines regulations, and health technology assessment, to increase the capacity of patients to understand and contribute to medicines research and development and even improve the availability of objective, reliable, patient-friendly information for the public. For this purpose, EUPATI provides several tools for the patients training such as the toolbox medicine development and English language patient expert training courses. EUPATI's interest in raising awareness of the clinical world on the patient empowerment has led to the launch of a public consultation, which ended in September 2016 with the release of the EUPATI guidance for patient involvement in the medicines research and development process [4]. Each guidance suggests an area where at present there are opportunities for patient involvement, and in particular:

- industry-led medicines R&D,
- ethical review of clinical trials,
- regulatory processes,
- health technology assessment (HTA).

The necessity to have a clear guidance on patient involvement in different areas of the medicines development process originates from some needs and lacks in the clinical research, such as:

- existing code of trial conduct does not describe the involvement of the patients,
- patients and patients' organizations should be involved proactively during early discovery, development, and postapproval stages and not only in the clinical development,
- overarching guidance on meaningful and ethical interaction is missing.

For these reasons, the guidance is devoted to provide recommendations for all stakeholders aiming to interact with patients, for example by delivering a clear and complete definition of "patient" (patients, carers/family representatives, expert patient advocates, etc.), establishing the operating procedures for a long-term interaction and explaining the key elements of a written collaboration agreement.

In particular, the guidance provides the following definitions:

- "**Individual patients**" are persons whose main contribution is represented by their personal experience of a disease or treatment regardless of whether they may or may not have specific knowledge in the medicine research and development process.
- With personal experience of living with a disease, they may or may not have technical knowledge in "**Carers**" who are paid or volunteer persons helping "individual patients."
- "**Patient advocates**" are persons who have knowledge and competences to gather patients living with a specific disease and to support them regardless if they may or may not be affiliated with an organization.
- "**Patient organization representatives**" are persons within a patient organization on a specific disease or issue, who have been designated to represent the point of view of the organization itself.
- "**Patient experts**" are patients with experience of living with a specific disease that, differently from "individual patients," have also specific knowledge in research and development

(R&D) and/or regulatory affairs achieved through training activities such as courses provided by EUPATI on the full spectrum of medicines R&D.

All these procedures are aimed to draw on patient knowledge and experience and understand what it is like to live with a specific condition, how care is administered, and the day-to-day use of the medicines. As a result, they allow to incorporate patient needs and priorities in an optimized drug development process as well as to achieve a constructive dialog with the patient and a functional exchange of information, fundamental to speed up a successful clinical process.

2.2. Summaries of clinical trial results for laypersons

On April 16, 2014, the European Parliament and the Council of the European Union (EU) released the Regulation EU No 536/2014 [5] on clinical trials on medicinal products for human use, to ensure that the rules for conducting clinical trials are identical through the EU. The aim of the Clinical Trial Regulation is to favor the conduction of the clinical trials in accordance with the highest standards of patient safety for all the EU Member States. These goals are achieved through some harmonized procedures for authorization, specific sponsor obligations, and simplified reporting procedures. Furthermore, such regulation foresees a section dedicated to communication of the results to patients. In particular, the article 37 requires sponsors to provide summary results of clinical trials in the EU Portal and Database in a format understandable to laypersons and the Annex V of the regulation outlines 10 elements that must be considered in the lay summary writing.

In this context, from June 1, 2016 to August 31, 2016, the Directorate General for Health and Food Safety, DG SANTE launched a public consultation on the "Summary of Clinical Trial Results for Laypersons," developed by the expert group on clinical trials, in order to collect comments and suggestions by all the stakeholders involved in clinical research to implement the Clinical Trials Regulation (EU) No 536/2014. The main objective of this document is to provide recommendations and templates for the production of a summary of clinical trial results for laypersons by sponsors and investigators, in accordance with Annex V of the EU Clinical Trials Regulation. Despite not mandatory, this document intends to make the summaries more accessible to the lay persons.

The **recommendations of the clinical trials expert group on the "Summaries of Clinical Trial Results for Laypersons"** [6], which have been published on January 2017 in EudraLex Volume 10, Chapter V, provide the following principles:

- develop the summary for a general public audience and do not assume any prior knowledge of the trial,
- develop the layout and content for each section in terms of style, language, and literacy level to meet the needs of the general public,
- keep the document as short as possible,
- focus on unambiguous, factual information,

- ensure that no promotional content is included,
- follow health literacy and numeracy principles, and
- consider involving patients, patient representatives, or advocates in the development and review of the summary information to ensure that it truly meets their needs.

In particular, the document provides detailed information about the health literacy level to consider in the summary, the readability specifying the size of the serif font, and the use of plain language, numeracy, and visuals. As the International Adult Literacy Survey identifies five levels of proficiency ranging from level 1 (lowest level) to level 5 (highest level), the document suggests that the text should be suitable for people with a low/medium average level of literacy (level 2 or 3). However, as readability scores are useful but not in themselves enough to ensure that a text is easy to understand, sponsors should consider, where feasible, testing the readability of an initial version of the study results' summary with a small number of people who represent the target population. Depending on the nature of the study, this could be patients with a particular disease or it could be members of the public. For example, studies, which affect the general public such as vaccine studies, would benefit from input from members of the public rather than patients. Their feedback and suggestions can be crucial in developing a summary that lay people will understand.

Moreover, the Annex I of the recommendations offers the templates with user-friendly equivalent headings, useful to prepare the summary, and even giving examples of wording more comprehensible for the target population.

Despite all attempts of increased awareness for the patient involvement in clinical research, rarely these initiatives pay attention to the pediatric population.

Children's active participation in the decision-making process is necessary not only in the daily clinical practice, but also and especially in all the activities related to the development and use of drugs. In the last years, the idea that children's preferences should always be taken into consideration is also agreed upon among parents. For this reason, healthcare professionals have to consider children and families' active participation as a fundamental step to reach consensus and compliance to treatments and research.

Furthermore, in 2012, following a large consultation phase, the Pediatric Committee (PDCO) issued a "concept paper on the involvement of children and young people" in its activities, with the children's best interests as primary consideration [7]. It has to be also highlighted that the setup of a child-friendly approach implies a collaborative and continuous action involving pediatricians and healthcare professionals, psychologists, families, and children.

Children and parents should be involved not only in the revision of clinical study protocols but also during the whole study development. Finally, it is necessary to recognize that a standard model of information is not valid for all age groups, above all for extreme groups.

2.3. Ethical considerations for clinical trials on medicinal products conducted with minors

The need to involve children actively in the decision-making process related to a clinical trial is clearly underlined also in the updating guideline "Ethical considerations for clinical trials on medicinal products conducted with minors" [8]. The document was released by a group chaired by the European Commission with the aim to develop guidelines to implement the Directive 2001/20/EC relating to good clinical practice in the conduct of clinical trials on medicinal products for human use. The document, opened for consultation from June to August 2016, provides recommendations on various ethical aspects of clinical trials performed in children from birth up to the legal age of adulthood and will contribute to the protection of all children who are the subject of clinical trials.

Moreover, it underlines that "the investigator and protocol writer should ensure that there is involvement of children (suffering from the relevant condition) and families in the development of informative material and where feasible, also in the design, analysis, and conduct of the trial." Consequently, even if the pediatric population is not specifically cited by the EU Clinical Trials Regulation 536/2014 (Article 37) requiring sponsors to provide summary results of clinical trials in a format understandable to laypersons, children cannot be excluded by the advantages of this obligation.

By definition, children (minors) are unable to consent (in the legal sense), but they should be involved in the process of informed consent as much as possible, using appropriate age information. In the ethical review, in fact, drawing on the pediatric expertise allows to balance the benefits, risks, and burden of research in minors. Moreover, the difference between minors and adults as research participants has implications on the design, conduct, and analysis of trials, which should also include pediatric expertise.

The Regulation EU 536/2014 provides a series of definitions in order to clarify some important concepts for the patient interaction and patient involvement and in particular the age groups. Defining the age range is necessary to have a guidance regarding the proper involvement of minors of different ages in the informed consent process. Subsets of the pediatric population as defined in ICH E11 (ICH Harmonized Tripartite Guideline—Clinical Investigation of Medicinal Products in the Pediatric Population E11) [9] are partially adopted, and the age groups of 2–11 years and 12–17 years have been redefined as follows:

- **preschoolers** (2–5 years)
- **schoolers** (6–9 years)
- **adolescents** (from the age of 10 up to but not including above 18 years)

Regardless of the age and with an appropriate communication, the clinical trial regulation states that the child should be involved in the process of informed consent. The article 2 of clinical trial regulation defines the "**Informed consent**" as the document expressing the will of a subject to participate in a particular clinical trial; the subject, after having received information on all the aspects of the clinical trial in which he/she will be involved, expresses his/her decision in a free and voluntary way. In case of minors and of incapacitated subjects, it is intended as an authorization or agreement from their legally designated representative to include them in the clinical trial [5].

Moreover, the article 29(8) of the clinical trials regulation adds that also a minor should assent firsthand to participate in the clinical trial in cases in which he/she is capable of forming an opinion and evaluating the information received, without prejudice to national law and in addition to the informed consent signed by the legally designated representative [5]. The ethical considerations document supports and highlights the legal value of the assent, suggesting that assent should be understood as a legally required expression of the minor's will to participate in a clinical trial, dependent on Member State law. According to this view, the assent should be considered in the same way as the consent of the parents/legally designated representative since it expresses with legal value the willingness of the child to participate in the clinical trial [8]. However, a minor who expresses the assent to join to a clinical trial cannot participate in it in absence of the informed consent signed by the parents/legally designated representative [8]. In addition, the consultation document introduces the term **agreement**, used in accordance with the term "assent," to describe the expression of will to participate in a clinical study given by the minor. The document also recommends systematically requiring the agreement when it is not legally mandatory and explains that the modalities to obtain it, in contrast to the legally required assent, are not age dependent but are related only to the [8]. If the minor is considered not mature enough to express his/her will to participate in a conscious manner, the lack of agreement does not necessarily mean the child will not participate in the clinical trial. However, dissent should be taken into due account in line with Article 32(1c) of the clinical trial regulation, when the minor, despite having proven his/her maturity, expresses his/her will not to participate [8].

Another important aspect discussed in the document is the importance to estimate to what extent a child is able to provide agreement. It is recommended to consider not only the chronological age, but also and especially **the developmental stage, intellectual capacities,** and **life/disease experiences** of the minor. The evaluation should be made after a careful discussion among the investigator, the parents/legally designated representative, and the child [8].

3. Patient and public involvement: the role of advocacy

Patient and public involvement (PPI) represents the active involvement of patients and/or individuals from the general population in scientific research with the aim to enhance quality and relevance of the research itself. Indeed, PPI strategies have shown in the last year to be key instruments to improve the conduction, the communication, and the prioritization of the research.

The involvement of service users in research has risen internationally, with patients' engagement in all the aspects of health and social care research. PPI plans have been included successfully in many clinical trial grant applications foreseeing patients' engagement in all the phases of clinical research: initial stages, undertaking phase, analysis and write-up, dissemination, and implementation [10].

Jo Brett et al. [11] carried out a systematic search of electronic databases and health libraries to identify the impact of PPI on health and social care research. The authors pointed out that PPI can have positive impact on research, enhancing its quality and ensuring its appropriateness and relevance. They also suggested that PPI strategies, to engage users in the initial stage of a medical research, are to be preferred since patients and lay people involvement in this step can shape the entire study and, users may have more freedom to influence the aims and methods of the study. Moreover, they underlined that a clear definition of the roles of all the professionals and users involved through a precise planning and procedure, and training activities are important factors determining the success of the PPI.

Also, challenges to the development of plans for PPI have been described including issues regarding their purpose, difficulties in ensuring sufficient resources and in the recruitment of service users, the long-term commitment needed from service users, and the time and cost limits imposed on studies. Nonetheless, all the challenges mentioned above can be avoided by a precise planning of the PPI strategy, especially in the early stage of a proposed study [10, 11].

Among the current policies to encourage public involvement, strategies based on the concept of advocacy are spreading all over the world.

The World Health Organization (WHO) gave a definition of Advocacy for Health in the Health Promotion Glossary published in 1998 as "a combination of individual and social actions designed to gain political commitment, policy support, social acceptance, and system support for a particular health goal or program" [1].

According to this definition, advocacy stands for acting or doing something to influence private and public policy choices' in order to achieve an individual or community objective.

Advocacy is one of the three strategies underpinning health promotion as described in the WHO Health Promotion Glossary mentioned above, and many strategies have been described to reach this goal including the use of the mass media and multimedia, direct political lobbying, and community mobilization through, for example, coalitions of interests around defined issues.

3.1. An innovative approach for the patient involvement: advisory groups in pediatric clinical research

When it comes to consider patient's involvement in the pediatric field, more challenges have to be faced since the engagement of children requires appropriate means and language and it is also necessary to take into due account all the relevant legal and ethical aspects.

Despite these challenges, children have the right to be involved and informed, to know in advance which medicines they need and why and to get access to the resulting evidence-based medicinal products. Their point of view has to be taken into due account in the design and planning of a clinical study, and they should be allowed to express their own views and granted the right to participate in the decision-making process concerning their own health.

An innovative approach for the patients' involvement in pediatric clinical research is represented by the **Young Persons Advisory Groups** widespread through the world. A Young Persons Advisory Group (YPAG) is an organization composed of youths, patients, carers, and people interested in a health condition or in research, actively participating as partners, advising researchers and their teams in a full range of activities in various research projects and initiatives.

After educational and training activities, the youths become able to help researchers in trial design, prioritizing future researches, improving communication with the target population, and increase awareness on clinical research through the different means of communication.

Many advisory groups have been founded, and all together they constitute the **International Children's Advisory Network (iCAN)** [12], a worldwide consortium of children's advisory groups or chapters working together to provide a voice for children and families in health, medicine, research, and innovation through synergy, communication, and collaboration. Within the consortium, various types of groups can be described, all working together for advocacy purposes in pediatric medicines:

- **Kids and families impacting disease through science, (KIDS)**: Advisory groups of children, adolescents, and families focused on understanding, communicating, and improving the process of medical innovation for children. KIDS groups have been created in Connecticut, Georgia, Missouri, Ohio, Illinois, Michigan, Texas, Florida, Barcelona, Australia, France, and recently in Italy and Albania.
- **Young Persons Advisory Groups**: a set-up in Great Britain (Liverpool, Birmingham, London, Bristol, and Nottingham) as Generation R [13] with the aim to increase the input and influence of children and their families or carers into the development of clinical research.
- **Kids Can** (Vancouver): promoting a direct engagement of young people in research and the **ScotCRN Young Persons Group** (Scotland) aimed to support clinical research to improve the safety and efficacy of children's medicines and healthcare.

Advocating for children in healthcare globally is the main purpose of the network as well as taking into due account the children and families' needs and willingness in health, research, medicine, and innovation in order to improve clinical research. iCAN's chapters work both locally in partnership with their local children's hospitals and communities and collaborate together network-wide to have a global impact.

Their slogan is: Together, we can improve the future of pediatric medicine!

The European chapters of iCAN (KIDS Barcelona, YPAG Birmingham, YPAG Bristol, KIDS France, YPAG Liverpool, YPAG London, YPAG Nottingham, YPAG Scotland) have recently established a **European YPAGs' network, or eYPAGnet** [14], under the coordination of Hospital Sant Joan de Déu (Barcelona) as part of the iCAN umbrella organization. This network arose from the need, recognized by the Enpr-EMA (European Network of Pediatric Research at the European Medicines Agency), to promote cooperation among European groups with the mission to improve the capacity of collaboration with the different actors who participate in the research and development process of innovative drugs in Europe.

Enpr-EMA has promoted several actions with the aim to foster engagement of young people and families in clinical research. A survey on the involvement of young people and family members in Enpr-EMA pediatric research networks was launched in August 2012 and highlighted that only three out of the 39 networks participating to the survey had developed strategies or guidelines for the involvement of young people and families. A second survey was conducted in November 2016 to investigate the point of view of the Pediatric Committee (PDCO) members in relation to the involvement of young people and families in the activities of the Committee. Moreover, a working group on young patient advisory groups has been established in order to develop harmonized procedures for a more European-oriented approach of YPAGs.

The working group has launched two surveys to investigate the characteristics of the existing YPAGs with the final aim to create a European network of young advisory groups and to define the best practices to address issues in the framework of the EU multilanguage YPAGs. Within these initiatives, eYPAGnet has been created and admitted, during 2017 annual meeting, as member of Enpr-EMA of category 4.

Among the main scopes of eYPAGnet, there are development of clinical research initiatives and empowerment training programs for children on a European level and the promotion of new chapters' set-up. Indeed, since June 2017, two new chapters, KIDS Bari and KIDS Albania have been created in Europe and are coordinated by Consorzio per Valutazioni Biologiche e Farmacologiche (CVBF) and the TEDDY Network (European Network of Excellence for Pediatric Clinical Research).

CVBF is a not-for-profit organization aimed to perform research in life science at European level with a special focus on drug development for small populations (pediatric and rare diseases). It provides scientific, economic, and regulatory consultancy in pediatric clinical research and a research management support in national and international research projects. Particular interest is given to promote educational activities supporting the consortium's areas of expertise and to favor knowledge and access to the results of biomedical research and accelerate their use by patients. The consortium has developed a considerable expertise in communication and dissemination field, leading and managing these activities in several EU-funded projects (GAPP, DEEP, CloSed, and InNerMeD).

The TEDDY Network was born as an EC-FP6-funded Network of Excellence (NoE) and now is an independent multidisciplinary and multinational network including 50 members in 20 EU and non-EU countries aimed to favor the integration of the pediatric pharmacological research activities, the implementation of adequate health policies, and a social awareness on the importance of the pediatric medicines across Europe covering different specialty areas (hematology, oncology, infectious diseases, respiratory diseases, intensive care, pain, endocrinology, rare diseases, neonatology, etc.).

TEDDY is a category 1 network member of Enpr-EMA and collaborates with existing pediatric networks and research organizations with the goal to promote and foster scientific and technological excellence in the pediatric research in Europe.

3.2. Advisory group contribution in pediatric clinical research

Existing advisory groups and initiatives have shown to be an effective form of patient and public involvement in the pediatric field providing fresh perspectives on pediatric clinical research and promoting changes of attitudes about the involvement of young people in all the aspects of medicines research.

The activities carried out by all the advisory groups across the world are aimed at contributing to raise awareness of the importance of patient and public involvement in the development of research trial.

The education and, in particular, the peer education is a fundamental aspect of the advocacy strategy. The **peer education** is an educational approach, recommended by modern development psychology, based on teaching and sharing information, values, and behavior relating to health promotion among lay people. Through this approach, advocacy groups aim to provide children and families with resources and opportunities to express their feedback and inputs about studies and products intended for children.

iCAN is a free resource available to any organization, company, or group, which seeks the input of children and families in their projects. iCAN chapters utilize online-based surveys, focus groups, forums, and more to engage all of the youth advisory groups in their network to provide specific feedback about clinical trials or any other process of medical innovation for children.

Moreover, many groups work on research projects on their own and participate in science conferences to disseminate their results and to highlight the importance of their involvement in research. Just to mention some examples of projects carried out by iCAN chapters, Kids Can developed a mobile application "Mobile Kids" [15] to encourage physical activity in kids aged between 8 and 13 years with the use of mobile technology.

Kids Can and Kids Connecticut participated in the development of guidelines aimed to standardize reporting of clinical trial protocol (SPIRIT-C) [16] and trial reports (CONSORT-C) [17] across pediatric studies.

Members of US, Canada, and UK young patients' advisory groups provided their contribution responding to a survey launched by the Global Alliance for Pediatric Therapeutics Assent Project [18], a project aimed to evaluate current practices, challenges, and unmet needs associated with the achievement of pediatric assent for clinical trials.

KIDS Barcelona group provided recommendations [19] to be taken into account by the sponsor of a clinical trial and ethics committee of the research center to make the assent form more understandable for children. The recommendations are collected in a guideline, available in Spanish and English, approved by iCAN and EUPATI and included in the guidelines for the design of a pediatric clinical trial by Agencia Española de Medicamentos y Productos Sanitarios (AEMPS). Moreover, the Spanish group has developed a series of eight different funny comics [20] to explain several matters of the clinical research using a language more familiar for the children.

Furthermore, YPAGs have given their useful contribution in the revision of informed consent/assent template prepared by Enpr-EMA within the activities of the working group 4 on ethics providing their thoughts and ideas to make the template more understandable by a wide range of ages.

By many activities and initiatives performed, the young advisor groups spread all over the world are able to help the professionals involved in the clinical trials to overcome some tough issues of the clinical research. For example, they could help to open and complete on time the trials or could improve the recruitment of patients to the agreed target and the retention of patients to completion. In general, through the YPAGs, the clinicians involved in the trials could meet the needs of the patients, designing the study according to their necessities.

4. Patient-centered approach to improve pediatric clinical research: some good practices

It is universally established that written communication, combined with verbal interaction, may enhance children's understanding of their participation in a clinical research [21] as well as the contents and styles of documents addressed to children are elements that largely influence their understanding of written documents.

As an example, it has been demonstrated that the use of pictures, following appropriate recommendations, improves the quality of communication, especially for patients with very low literacy skills. However, available data and publications show that ad hoc informative strategies for empowering minors in clinical trials are rarely produced. In addition, the difficulty increases in multicenter trials, involving countries with different cultural and educational backgrounds.

This is the assumption at the basis of the development of age-tailored information booklets, assent forms, and videos prepared in the framework of the DEferiprone Evaluation in Pediatrics [22] (DEEP) and GAbapentin in Pediatric Pain [23] (GAPP) projects, two EC-FP7 funded projects coordinated by Consorzio per Valutazioni Biologiche e Farmacologiche (CVBF).

All the materials have been developed with a language and a wording appropriate to age, psychological and intellectual maturity, taking into account the cultural and linguistic differences, in a collaborative effort among pharmacologists, pediatricians, child psychologists, and illustrators.

In the framework of the GAPP project, aimed to confirm the efficacy and safety of gabapentin in pediatric patients affected by chronic pain with a neuropathic component, three booklets and two videos (**Figure 2**) have been created to inform the child participant on the study objectives and procedures. Two assent forms have been released to obtain his/her consent to

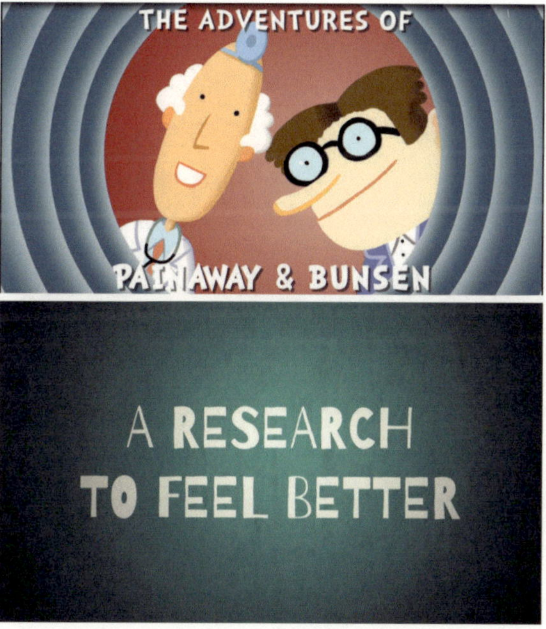

Figure 2. GAPP projects' video: in the framework of the GAPP project activities, two videos have been developed to inform the child participant on the study objectives and procedures according to two age ranges (for children on the top and for teenagers on the bottom).

Jack and Sarah have got anemia.
This year they want to find out whether Doctor Ironless's new syrup works as well as the tablets do.
Once a week they go to the hospital.
Nora the nurse takes a sample of their blood.
Once a month, they have an appointment with Doctor Ironless.
At home, Sarah takes the syrup three times a day.
Jack takes one tablet every day, dissolved in water.
At the end of the year, the doctor will find out whether he can give his new syrup to other children.
Do you want to be like Jack and Sarah?
metrodeep
Your route, step by step
Syrup
Tablets
Electrocardiogram
Check-up
Blood sample
Questionnaire
Magnetic resonance imaging of the heart and the liver
ARRIVAL
START
THE RULES FOR OUR TRIAL
344 children and young people under the age of 18
14 months of trial
6 days without any medicine
12 months with the syrup or soluble tablets
Remember:
At the beginning of the trial, doctors will pick the children's names out of a hat and divide them into two groups. The first group will take the syrup and the second group will take the tablets.
Jump onto the track to find out what you will be doing each month!
GO!
ONE month later
FINISH
= soluble tablets
= syrup
= 4 samples per month
= medical check-up
= in-depth check-up
During the trial, some children will do more tests on their heart and liver. But no worries: these tests are very simple!

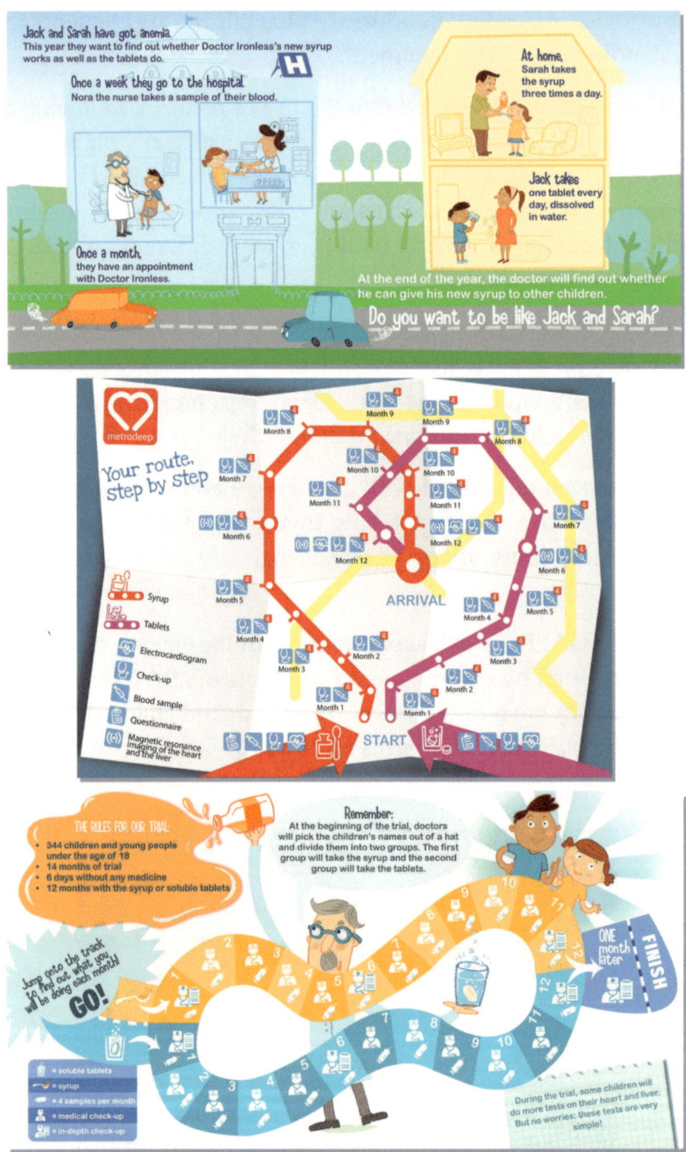

Figure 3. DEEP project booklets: the pages extracted from the three booklets, developed for three different age ranges (age range 0–6, 6–10, and 10–17, respectively, in the top, middle, and bottom pages), explain how the clinical trial will be carried out.

participate in the study. A patient diary has also been developed to register specific daily data on the use of the Investigational Medicinal Products (IMPs), rescue and concomitant medication, pain scores, and adverse effects when the patient is at home. It also contains instructions for the use of the IMP, troubleshooting, and contact details of the study's medical staff.

For the young participants of the DEEP project, aimed to marketing a new formulation of deferiprone for the treatment of iron overload in pediatric patients affected by congenital anemia, three different booklets (**Figure 3**) explaining clinical trial aims and procedures and what they are going to experience, and two different assent forms were prepared. For both projects, all these informative materials are available in all the languages of the project.

Informative videos (a spoonful of info helps the medicine go down) [24], specifically addressed to children between 4 and 7 years old explaining some main concepts on drugs and their use, have also been developed by the TEDDY Network of Excellence for Pediatric Clinical Research within the empowerment activities addressed to young patients in the healthcare field.

5. Conclusions

There is a need to change attitudes in order to make the patients' empowerment a priority in the clinical research field. Patients have to take an active role in activities or decisions that will have consequences for the patient community, because of their specific knowledge and relevant experience as patients. Children's active participation in the decision-making process is needed not only in the daily clinical practice, but also in all the activities related to the development and use of drugs. Minor shall take part in the informed consent procedure in a way adapted to his/her age and mental maturity.

Patients/families need to be considered as "co-managers" of their condition and participate in decisions related to their healthcare according to their capacity. Moreover, patients (individually and) collectively have to play a role in improving healthcare services for all patients by contributing with their specific experiences as learning and educational tools to inform and (re-) design of services.

However, the involvement must be planned, appropriately resourced, carried out, and evaluated as to its outcomes, impact, and the process itself, according to the values and purposes of all participants. Engaging children early in the research process and educating the world about the importance of participating in clinical research could increase the level of participation in pediatric clinical trials, thus reducing the patients' retention and fostering treatment compliance. Moreover, a patient-centered approach can improve the capacity of collaboration with the different agents, who participate in the research process and in the development of innovative drugs.

Author details

Mariangela Lupo[1,2]*, Angelica Intini[1] and Doriana Filannino[1]

*Address all correspondence to: mlupo@cvbf.net

1 CVBF – Consorzio per le Valutazioni Biologiche e Farmacologiche, Bari, Italy

2 TEDDY – European Network of Excellence for Paediatric Clinical Research, Pavia, Italy

References

[1] WHO Health Promotion Glossary. 1998. Available from: http://www.who.int/healthpromotion/about/HPR%20Glossary%201998.pdf

[2] Angelmar R, Bermann BP. Patient empowerment and efficient health outcomes. Financing Sustainable Healthcare in Europe. 2007:139-162

[3] EUPATI. Official Website. Dec 1, 2016. Available from: https://www.eupati.eu/

[4] EUPATI. Guidance Documents on Patient Involvement in R&D. Dec 14, 2016. Available from: https://www.eupati.eu/guidance-patient-involvement/

[5] Regulation (EU) No 536/2014 of the European Parliament and of the Council of 16 April 2014 on clinical trials on medicinal products for human use, and repealing Directive 2001/20/EC. Apr 16, 2014. Available from: https://ec.europa.eu/health/sites/health/files/files/eudralex/vol-1/reg_2014_536/reg_2014_536_en.pdf

[6] Summaries of Clinical Trial Results for Laypersons. Recommendations of the Expert Group on Clinical Trials for the Implementation of Regulation (EU) No 536/2014 on Clinical Trials on Medicinal Products for Human Use. Jan 26, 2017. Available from: https://ec.europa.eu/health/sites/health/files/files/eudralex/vol-10/2017_01_26_summaries_of_ct_results_for_laypersons.pdf

[7] EMA Concept Paper on the Involvement of Children and Young People at the Paediatric Committee (PDCO). Sep 17, 2012. Available from: http://www.ema.europa.eu/docs/en_GB/document_library/Scientific_guideline/2012/09/WC500132555.pdf

[8] Ethical Considerations for Clinical Trials on Medicinal Products Conducted with Minors. Recommendations of the Expert Group on Clinical Trials for the Implementation of Regulation (EU) No 536/2014 on Clinical Trials on Medicinal Products for Human Use. Jun 2, 2016. Available from: https://ec.europa.eu/health//sites/health/files/files/clinicaltrials/2016_06_pc_guidelines/gl_1_consult.pdf

[9] ICH Harmonised Tripartite Guideline. Clinical Investigation of Medicinal Products in the Pediatric Population. E11. Nov 15, 2005 Available from: http://www.ich.org/fileadmin/Public_Web_Site/ICH_Products/Guidelines/Efficacy/E11/Step4/E11_Guideline.pdf

[10] Buck D, Gamble C, Dudley L, et al. From plans to actions in patient and public involvement: Qualitative study of documented plans and the accounts of researchers and patients sampled from a cohort of clinical trials. BMJ Open. 2014;**4**:e006400. DOI: 10.1136/bmjopen-2014-006400

[11] Brett J, Staniszewska S, Mockford C, Herron-Marx S, Hughes J, Tysall C, Suleman R. Mapping the impact of patient and public involvement on health and social care research: A systematic review. Health Expectations. Oct 2014;**17**(5):637-650. DOI: 10.1111/j.1369-7625.2012.00795.x [Epub Jul 19, 2012]. Review. PubMed PMID: 22809132; PubMed Central PMCID: PMC5060910

[12] iCAN Official Website. Dec 28, 2016. Available from: https://icanresearch.org

[13] Generation R Official Website. May 10, 2015. Available from: http://generationr.org.uk/about/

[14] KIDS Barcelona Official Website. Jan 18, 2017. Available from: https://www.kidsbarcelona.org/en/eypagnet

[15] KidsCan Young Persons Advisory Group webpage. Dec 18, 2014. Available from: http://bcchr.ca/kidscan/mobilekids

[16] SPIRIT-C Project Webpage. Nov 28, 2013. Available from: http://www.sickkids.ca/Research/EnRICH/Research-Projects-and-Initiatives/SPIRIT-C/index.html

[17] CONSORT-C Project Webpage. Nov 28, 2013. Available from: http://www.sickkids.ca/Research/EnRICH/Research-Projects-and-Initiatives/CONSORT-C/index.html

[18] Global Alliance for Paediatric Therapeutics Webpage. May 18, 2016. Available from: http://www.pediatricinnovation.org/drug-reformulation/

[19] Guidelines for a Design Focused on the Children are Available at the KIDS Barcelona Official Website. Jan 18, 2017. Available from: https://www.kidsbarcelona.org/sites/default/files/aaff_eupati_english.pdf

[20] Comics are Available at the KIDS Barcelona Official Website. Jan 18, 2017. Available from: https://www.kidsbarcelona.org/sites/default/files/comic_ensayos_clinicos.pdf

[21] Ungar D, Joffe S, Kodish E. Children are not small adults: Documentation of assent for research involving children. The Journal of Pediatrics. 2006;**149**:s31-ss3

[22] DEEP Official Website. Sep 02, 2017 Available from: https://www.deepproject.eu/

[23] GAPP Official Website. May 26, 2017. Available from: https://www.pediatricpain.eu/

[24] TEDDY Videos are Available at the TEDDY Official Website. Feb 15, 2017. Available from: https://www.teddynetwork.net/teddy-videos-drug-use-explained-to-children/

Section 3

Clinical Trials on Stem Cell Therapy

Chapter 4

Unique Aspects of the Design of Phase I/II Clinical Trials of Stem Cell Therapy

Ivonne H. Schulman, Wayne Balkan,
Russell Saltzman, Daniel DaFonseca, Lina V. Caceres,
Cindy Delgado, Marietsy V. Pujol, Kevin N. Ramdas,
Jairo Tovar, Mayra Vidro-Casiano and
Joshua M. Hare

Additional information is available at the end of the chapter

http://dx.doi.org/10.5772/intechopen.72949

Abstract

This chapter will review the unique aspects and limitations of the design of phase I/II (safety and efficacy) clinical trials of stem cell therapy. Although the classical pharmacologic principles applicable to drugs are not applicable to biologic (live cell) therapeutic agents, an important stage in the development of any new therapeutic agent is the establishment of an optimal dosage and delivery route. This can be particularly challenging when the treatment is a biologic agent, such as stem cells, that may exert its therapeutic effects via complex or poorly understood mechanisms. To date, clinical studies have shown inconsistent findings regarding the relationship between cell dose and clinical outcomes. This can be at least partially attributed to variations in donor cell type, source, characteristics, dosing/concentration, delivery route, underlying mechanisms of action, and efficacy endpoints tested. The current recommendations will be reviewed herein to give new investigators a general understanding of the unique issues that need to be considered and addressed when designing a stem cell therapy phase I/II clinical trial.

Keywords: phase I/II clinical trial, regenerative medicine, stem cells

1. Introduction

The past decade has witnessed the exciting development of novel stem cell therapies aimed at regenerating or restoring organ function. Preclinical and pilot studies using stem cells derived from a variety of tissue sources have led to the conduct of phase I/II clinical trials for chronic diseases, formerly thought to be incurable. Systems currently targeted for stem cell therapy

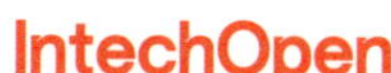

include cardiovascular, neurologic, pulmonary, autoimmune and liver diseases, as well as diabetes, frailty, and cutaneous wounds, among others [1–20]. In cardiovascular diseases, preclinical studies have served to provide feasibility, safety, and, importantly, mechanistic insights [21–27], whereas phase I/II studies have provided evidence, in the short-term, of the safety and efficacy of autologous and allogeneic bone marrow-derived mesenchymal stem cells (MSCs) [1, 2, 6, 18, 28, 29], autologous bone marrow and peripheral CD34+ stem cells [30, 31], and autologous cardiac-derived stem cells [32–34] in humans. Nevertheless, studies are lacking comparing the efficacy and sustainability of the various different cell types, as well as identifying the most effective dose, time of delivery, and route of administration. Other important questions that remain to be investigated are whether concurrent pharmacologic treatments beneficially or adversely interact with the various cell therapies and whether cell therapy increases the risk for opportunistic infections or malignancy development or progression [27, 35, 36]. Only through the rigorous conduct of large, multicenter clinical trials that include well-defined clinical endpoints and outcomes, a longer duration of follow up (years) and larger number of patients can these questions be addressed [37]. Of note, new biological therapeutic strategies, such as stem cell therapy, necessitates new evaluations tools that elucidate mechanisms of action and measure clinically relevant outcomes. From cell type to dosing, timing, and delivery as well as evaluating safety and clinical efficacy, stem cell therapy provides both unique opportunities and challenges in our quest to develop effective and sustainable therapeutic strategies for cardiovascular diseases as well as other chronic and disabling conditions [37].

Successful stem cell based therapy involves a complex orchestration of events, including engraftment and differentiation as well as secretion of bioactive molecules that inhibit apoptosis and fibrosis and stimulate neovascularization and endogenous stem cell recruitment, proliferation, and differentiation [35, 38, 39]. Notably, existing mechanistic studies support the importance of cell–cell interactions between MSCs and host cells within stem cell niches, which provide structural support and produce the soluble signals that regulate stem cell function in tissues [21, 24, 25, 39, 40]. This enhanced phenotypic and mechanistic understanding of the underpinnings of stem cell based therapy can be harnessed for improved clinical trial design as well as for development of newer generations of cellular as well as new molecular products that have greater efficacy and sustainability [36, 37].

This chapter will provide a general understanding of the unique issues that need to be considered and addressed when designing a phase I/II (safety and efficacy) stem cell therapy clinical trial for cardiovascular disease. The concepts are applicable to other chronic diseases for which stem cell therapeutic approaches are being developed and investigated [19]. For instance, the use of cells as therapeutic agents differs in significant ways from the established principles of pharmacokinetics and pharmacodynamics utilized in pharmacology. An important stage in the development of any new therapeutic agent is the establishment of an optimal dose and route of administration [29, 36]. Biologic therapies create unique challenges in this regard because they exert their therapeutic effects via complex or undefined mechanisms. Indeed, although clinical trials of stem cell therapy for various diseases began over a decade ago, specification of optimal dosage and delivery has not been established. The available clinical studies have shown inconsistent findings regarding the relationship

http://dx.doi.org/10.5772/intechopen.72949

between cell dose and clinical benefit, due, at least in part, to variations in donor cell characteristics, cell types, cell dosing/concentration, and route (intravenous, intra-arterial, intra-tissue) and timing of administration [29, 36]. We will also review the unique aspects of the selection of clinically relevant endpoints, donors and donor cell characteristics, and autologous versus allogeneic cell therapy.

2. Description and regulatory aspects

The customary first-in-human study or phase 1 investigation is used to determine the dose and timing of an investigational drug or biologic agent, as well as identify adverse events associated with agent administration in a dose-dependent fashion. Prior to designing a phase I study, it is critical that appropriate preclinical studies are conducted. Moreover, the clinical study must be conducted with appropriate ethical and quality standards, which includes protocol approval by the institutional review board (IRB), also known as an independent ethics committee (IEC), ethical review board (ERB), or research ethics board (REB). These committees review the methods proposed for the research study and monitor the study, in parallel with the data safety monitoring board (DSMB), for adherence to the protocol and adverse event reporting throughout the study period until completion. An important goal of a standard phase I clinical trial is to determine the maximally tolerated dose and/or recommended dose for further testing in larger phase II efficacy trials. Phase II studies aim to provide further information on dosing, tolerability, and major safety concerns, and potential for efficacy in the target patient population. These data are then utilized by researchers and sponsors to estimate the chance of success in achieving important clinical endpoints, such as mortality and hospitalization risk reduction, in phase III trials, obtain drug approval by the regulatory agencies, and bring the intervention into the market for use by clinicians as standard of care.

In the United States, in order to obtain approval, sponsors of drugs or biologic products not previously authorized for marketing in the United States must submit an Investigational New Drug (IND) application to the Food and Drug Administration (FDA) [41]. IND applications must contain sufficient information about the drug or biologic agent, investigators, clinical protocol, and nonclinical toxicologic data. Safety and efficacy must be supported by evidence from controlled studies of adequate size with disease-appropriate endpoints. The conventional approach to obtaining favorable consideration for a marketing license for a new drug or biologic agent is to do 2 or more large scale clinical trials designed to establish clinical benefit directly, often including a comparison between the new drug and a control drug to show improvement in survival, quality of life, or an existing surrogate endpoint for one of the outcomes.

At the time of submission of an IND or as an amendment to an existing IND, a request for regenerative medicine advanced therapy (RMAT) designation can be made. The twenty-first Century Cures Act describes the criteria required for RMAT designation (www.FDA.gov). According to the FDA, the criteria include that, (a) "the drug be a regenerative medicine therapy, which is defined as a cell therapy, therapeutic tissue engineering product, human cell and tissue product, or any combination product using such therapies or products, except for those regulated solely under Section 361 of the Public Health Service Act and part 1271 of Title 21, Code of Federal Regulations"; (b) "the drug is intended to treat, modify, reverse, or cure a serious or life-threatening disease or condition"; and (c) "preliminary clinical evidence indicates that the drug has the potential to address unmet medical needs for such disease or condition" (www.FDA.gov).

The process of obtaining an IND usually requires many years and vast financial resources. As part of the 1997 FDA Modernization Act, three fast-track FDA approval programs were enacted into law to allow for accelerated approval of certain eligible agents. The FDA fast-track program reduced the review period needed to bring first-in class agents to market and quickened the approval of agents that combat serious or life-threatening illnesses that lack standard treatments. With this addition of alternative paths to marketing approval that eased some of the stringent FDA requirements, designing proper phase I trials became even more important to help make early decisions about the potential efficacy of a drug or biologic agent.

The FDA Amendments Act of 2007 (FDAAA) reviewed, expanded, and reaffirmed several existing pieces of legislation regulating the FDA. These changes allowed the FDA to perform more comprehensive reviews of potential new drugs and devices. The FDAAA extended the authority to levy fees to companies applying for approval of drugs, expanded clinical trial guidelines for pediatric drugs, and created the priority review voucher program to expedite the review process for drugs that are expected to have a particularly great impact on the treatment of a disease. The program grants a voucher for use of priority review to a drug developer as an incentive to develop treatments for neglected diseases. The voucher can be used for future drugs that could have wider indications for use, but the company is required to pay a fee to use the voucher. The FDA Safety and Innovation Act of 2012 (FDASIA) is a piece of regulatory legislation that provides the FDA the authority to collect user fees from the medical industry to fund reviews of innovator drugs, medical devices, generic drugs, and biosimilar biologics. It also created the breakthrough therapy designation program and extended the priority review voucher program to make rare pediatric diseases eligible. Breakthrough therapy was designed to further expedite drug development, and was not meant to require that the drug be an actual "breakthrough" [42]. The goal was to facilitate and prioritize the FDA review of new drugs for serious or life-threatening diseases for which early phase clinical trials demonstrated significant treatment benefits over the existing therapeutic options [41].

Another critical regulatory aspect of the design and implementation of a clinical trial is ensuring subject protection and data quality to make certain that the study and its conclusions are robust and can support future trials as well as potential regulatory submissions for marketing approval. Good clinical practice (GCP) is the internationally recognized quality standard used to maintain safeguards on quality, safety, and efficacy. GCP represents ethical and scientific quality standards for designing, recording, and reporting trials that involve the participation of human subjects. Successful implementation of GCP reduces or obviates the need to duplicate the testing carried out during the research and development of novel agents. The International Council for Harmonization of Technical Requirements provides guidelines for GCP for Pharmaceuticals for Human Use (ICH). This is a project that assembles the regulatory authorities and pharmaceutical industry experts of Europe, Japan and the United States to review and deliberate the scientific and technical aspects of pharmaceutical product registration [43]. The mission and goal of the ICH is to streamline the research and development of new treatments by minimizing or removing testing duplication and producing greater harmonization in the interpretation and application of technical guidelines and requirements for product registration. The process of harmonization aims to develop a more efficient use of human, small and large animal, and material resources and to accelerate the global development and availability of new therapeutic strategies. Importantly, this needs to be achieved without reducing quality, safety, and efficacy and regulatory obligations to protect public health. The ICH guidelines have been adopted as law in several countries, but in the United States they remain only as guidance for the FDA [43].

As part of GCP, a detailed data safety and monitoring plan is implemented for all clinical trials. The plan should include a reporting system to the data coordinating center (DCC) as well as to the independent data and safety monitoring board (DSMB). The DSMB is tasked with the responsibility for safeguarding the interests of study participants, assessing the safety and efficacy of study procedures, and for monitoring the overall conduct of the trial. Web-based computing systems for data collection and data management must be compliant with current federal regulations, specifically, Title 21 of the CFR parts 210–211 (GMP), 820 (Quality System Regulation for Medical Devices), and 11 (Electronic Records and Electronic Signatures). Electronic Case Report Forms (eCRFs) are used to capture the data appropriate to address study objectives by the DCC. The clinical trial coordinators undergo the appropriate training by the DCC in order to have continuous access to enrollment, randomization, and data submission. Randomization for the clinical trials is performed centrally by the DCC. For stem cell clinical trials, a randomized treatment assignment is generated and sent to the study team and cell-manufacturing laboratory. The protocol coordinator, through regular site visits, monitors the quality and timeliness of data submission, as well as compliance with the study protocol, and works with the clinical center to address any deficiencies or discrepancies. A site visit report is distributed to the investigative team and the trial's sponsoring agency. In regard to adverse events (AE), standard operating procedures (SOPs) are developed that outline the reporting requirements for both the FDA and DSMB. For example, automatic emails are generated each time an AE is reported and serious adverse events (SAEs) require an independent medical monitor review that is located at the DCC. Back-up mechanisms are employed in the form of a weekly summary that is provided to the safety and regulatory group to ensure that the AEs receive the proper attention. If an AE requires expedited reporting to the FDA or the DSMB, the DCC prepares a detailed report based on the medical monitor's adjudication and source documentation received by the center. DCCs normally have internal tracking mechanisms to ensure meeting regulatory reporting requirements and to document DSMB responses.

Stem cell therapy clinical trials require a good manufacturing practice (GMP) cell manufacturing facility. These facilities are accredited by the foundation for the accreditation of cellular therapy (FACT). The GMP facilities are expected to have a Quality Assurance (QA) team that is responsible for the documentation system. This typically includes the Standard Operating Procedures (SOP) documents, Certificates of Analysis, documents with specifications for critical materials, supplies, and reagents, and master batch production records. The GMP facility is expected to have cell-manufacturing rooms that are supplied with all the necessary equipment, such as biosafety cabinets, incubators, bench top centrifuges, and microscopes. The laboratories in the facility must be HEPA filtered, under appropriate air handling (positive pressure), and must meet class 10,000 specifications in the manufacturing rooms and class 100,000 in the general laboratory, liquid nitrogen freezer rooms, storage rooms, and gown in/out areas. Standard operating procedures require that all laboratory equipment is cleaned and maintained according to established quality control schedules. Internal and external audits of the quality systems ensure compliance with current FDA requirements (21 CFR Part 1271 & 21 CFR Part 210 & 211) and other applicable standards from AABB, FACT, and JCAHO (CLIA). The goal of the comprehensive quality systems is to monitor the daily operational and manufacturing activities of the GMP facility in order to prevent, detect and correct flaws or inadequacies that could adversely impact the safety of patients and/or the safety, purity, potency, or efficacy of the manufactured cell therapy products.

3. Limitations of phase I/II trials of stem cell therapy for CVD

3.1. Cell types

Various different cell types are currently undergoing investigation in phase I/II clinical trials, including mesenchymal stem cells, cardiac-derived stem or progenitor cells, and bone marrow derived mononuclear cells. The cell characteristics, secretomes, and mechanisms of action of these various stem cells are under intense investigation but have not been completely elucidated. The modes of delivery utilized also vary according to the specific disease process and these include intravenous, intracoronary, and intramyocardial or transendocardial [27, 36], as will be discussed in a separate section.

Growing evidence shows the potential of bone marrow derived MSCs as a safe, durable, sustainable, and novel cell-based biologic therapeutic for a diverse range of clinical applications aimed at preventing or reversing organ injury and promoting tissue regeneration. There are numerous advantages to using MSCs as a therapeutic strategy. MSCs are relatively easy to isolate and expand; they exhibit multilineage differentiation capacity, immunomodulatory, anti-inflammatory, anti-fibrotic, and trophic effects; they home to injury sites; and they have an excellent safety profile in both autologous and allogeneic transplantation [2, 6, 8, 21, 22, 44, 45]. Importantly, the use of MSCs engenders few ethical issues since they originate from adult tissues. Preclinical models employing large animals have been instrumental in advancing phenotypic and mechanistic insights underlying MSC therapy for heart disease [21–24]. Furthermore, the growing human phenotypic data supports the notion that MSC therapy is safe [1, 2, 8, 18, 19, 46] and has the capacity for repair of diverse organ systems and amelioration of multiple disease processes [1–17, 19, 29]. The field is advancing rapidly and numerous MSC sources, including bone marrow, adipose tissue, umbilical cord blood, umbilical cord, and amniotic membranes/placenta are under investigation. Successful MSC therapy involves a complex orchestration of events, including MSC engraftment, differentiation, and, perhaps more importantly, secretion of bioactive molecules that inhibit apoptosis and fibrosis and stimulate neovascularization and endogenous stem cell recruitment, proliferation, and differentiation [35, 38]. Notably, existing mechanistic studies support the importance of cell–cell interactions between MSCs and host cells within stem cell niches, which provide structural support and produce the soluble signals that regulate stem cell function in tissues [21, 24]. This enhanced phenotypic and mechanistic understanding of the underpinnings of MSC-based therapy can be harnessed for improved clinical trial design as well as for development of newer generations of MSC products that have greater efficacy and sustainability.

Cardiac-derived stem or progenitor cells are adult resident multipotent stem cell population(s) identified by characteristic cell markers, including c-kit (CD117), sca-1, Isl1, and Wilms tumor 1, and by the ability to form cardiospheres in vitro [47–49]. Substantial evidence demonstrates that cardiac stem cells (CSCs) reside in stem cell niches in the heart and not only participate in myocardial homeostasis but also proliferate and differentiate in response to myocardial injury [21, 49, 50]. CSCs can differentiate into cardiomyocyte, endothelial, and smooth muscle cell lineages [49, 51, 52], although their degree of contribution to the generation of new cardiomyocytes is controversial [52–55]. Despite ongoing controversy [53–55], multiple preclinical studies, including a recent meta-analysis [56], have demonstrated that injection of CSCs into animal models of ischemic heart disease slowed the progression of pathological cardiac structural changes and improved cardiac function [24, 25, 49, 56–59].

Phase I/II clinical trials are building upon these promising preclinical results. Bolli and colleagues demonstrated the safety and efficacy of c-kit + autologous CSCs in patients with heart failure scheduled to undergo Coronary Artery Bypass Graft surgery [32, 60, 61]. With regards to efficacy, the study showed improvement in cardiac function as well as reduction in myocardial infarct size at the 4-month and 1 year time points. Takehara and colleagues evaluated the safety and therapeutic efficacy of autologous CSCs in combination with a sustained release hydrogel matrix producing a controlled release of basic fibroblast growth factor (bFGF) to augment the effect of the cells in patients with heart failure due to ischemic heart disease [62]. This study demonstrated that tissue engineering offers the potential to improve the poor cell survival post-injection, one of the major obstacles limiting the effectiveness of cell therapy, irrespective of the cell type.

The other major cardiac-derived cell therapy currently under clinical investigation is the "cardiosphere." Cardiospheres are undifferentiated cells isolated from subcultures of atrial or ventricular biopsy specimens. They grow as self-adherent clusters [47] and have been described as clonogenic, expressing stem and endothelial progenitor cell markers, and having properties of adult cardiac stem cells, including long-term self-renewal and differentiation into cardiomyocyte (demonstrating contractile activity and/or expressing cardiomyocyte markers), endothelial, and smooth muscle cell lineages in vitro and in vivo [47]. Cardiospheres are a mixture of both early-stage committed and primitive cells, comprised of a core of c-kit + stem cells, layers of differentiating cells, and an outer cell layer of mesenchymal stromal cells [48]. Preclinical models demonstrate that cardiosphere-derived cells (CDCs) are able to reduce scar size after myocardial infarction, improve cardiac function, and increase the viability of myocardium [63]. A Phase I clinical trial of autologous CDCs delivered by intracoronary infusion in patients with impaired cardiac function 2–4 weeks after myocardial infarction demonstrated both cell safety and cell efficacy, reported as increased viable myocardium, improved regional contractility, and reduced scar mass post treatment [34].

Bone marrow is a source of heterogeneous stem cells and progenitors that have the capacity to differentiate into various cell lineages. Clinical trials employing autologous bone marrow mononuclear cells (BM-MNCs) have evaluated the impact of timing of cell delivery after acute myocardial infarction [64–69]. Although BM-MNC therapy has repeatedly been shown to be safe, delivery in the immediate environment and up to 4 weeks after myocardial infarction has not been consistently or conclusively effective for improving cardiac function or structure.

In patients with chronic ischemic heart failure, a phase II trial investigated the efficacy of transendocardial delivery of BM-MNCs on cardiac performance and perfusion at 6 months [70]. Although the study showed no significant effect on cardiac structural or functional parameters, exploratory (post-hoc) analyses demonstrated significant improvement in cardiac function that was associated with higher counts of bone marrow $CD34^+$ and $CD133^+$ progenitor cells. These findings suggest that the bone marrow's cellular composition dictates clinical efficacy and that specific cell populations yield a larger regenerative benefit [71].

BM-MNCs have also been tested in clinical trials of refractory angina, a condition characterized by frequent angina attacks unresponsive to maximal medical therapy, and obstructive coronary artery disease not amenable to coronary revascularization [72]. A recent meta-analysis found that cell-based therapy produces improvement in measures of cardiac function and use of anti-anginal medications, and a decreased risk of major adverse cardiovascular events [73]. Notably, an improvement in myocardial perfusion, assessed by single photon emission computed tomography (SPECT), was also noted and there were significantly fewer atrial and ventricular arrhythmias in the cell therapy group. Previous meta-analyses [74, 75] reported similar results of decreased angina frequency and myocardial infarction rate and improved exercise tolerance.

Together the above clinical trials established the safety profile of the BM-MNCs in acute myocardial infarction, chronic ischemic heart failure, and refractory angina. Some of these trials [67–69] also emphasized the need to further optimize clinical trials with the goal of determining the ideal therapeutic time, cell administration route, cell population, and cell dose after acute myocardial infarction [36]. It is worth noting that two meta-analyses [76, 77] provided evidence of efficacy, indicating that BM-MNC therapy prevents pathologic cardiac structural changes, which continue during long-term follow-up, specifically by decreasing infarct size and left ventricular enlargement. In addition, one of these meta-analyses reported that administration of BM-MNCs in patients with ischemic heart disease reduced mortality, recurrent myocardial infarction, and stent thrombosis.

Collectively, the multiple clinical trials using BM-MNCs suggest that despite the benefits of easy accessibility, ability to obtain large quantity of cells without a need for ex vivo expansion, vast preclinical and clinical bone marrow transplantation experience, and a positive safety profile [76, 77], there are significant concerns regarding the efficacy of BM-MNCs for acute myocardial infarction and chronic ischemic heart failure [1, 67, 68, 70]. It is important to note that these completed phase I trials were primarily focused on establishing the safety profile of BM-MNCs, and efficacy results may have been limited by the small number of patients. The multicenter, randomized, controlled, phase III study entitled "The Effect of Intracoronary Reinfusion of BM-MNC on All Cause Mortality in Acute Myocardial Infarction (BAMI) trial" (NCT01569178) is designed to test efficacy and is currently ongoing.

3.2. Donors and donor cell characteristics: age, comorbidities, carcinogenic potential, and sex differences

The proper use of stem cells for clinical applications requires a general understanding of the stem cell aging process [78]. For instance, as MSCs age, their multilineage differentiation, homing, immune modulation and wound healing properties gradually become compromised [78, 79]. Indeed, aging has detrimental effects on stem cells [78, 80, 81], with recent evidence suggesting a "quiescence-to-senescence switch" [82]. These age-related declines in stem cell therapeutic efficiency may be due to intrinsic stem cell aging and age-related changes in the local (tissue) environment, including extracellular matrix components and the stem cell niche [81, 83, 84]. Together these changes produce a decline in stem cell self-renewal, maintenance and therapeutic potential. Thus, the ability of MSCs to function therapeutically likely depends on the age and health status of the donor.

Although the effects of aged MSCs on cardiac repair have not been measured directly, studies have compared the effects of age and comorbidities on human bone marrow cell "angiogenic potency." Aging, renal failure, C-reactive protein and other health factors correlated significantly with poor angiogenic potency of bone marrow cells [85, 86]. Similarly, the number and migratory capacity of endothelial progenitor cells was reduced in hypertensive patients [87] and those suffering with ischemic cardiomyopathy [88]. Extrapolating these findings to stem-cell therapy for heart disease, suggests that the therapeutic potential of autologous MSCs obtained from patients with ischemic heart disease would allow for only limited recovery, whereas a more robust cardiac repair would occur if allogeneic MSCs from young, healthy donors were used instead. However, while it seems that age and/or comorbidities have a negative impact on the cardiac therapeutic potential of MSCs, such a direct comparison has not been conducted. Alternatively, a study on recipient age and stem cell therapy by Golpanian et al. showed that older (>60 years old) patients respond just as effectively as younger (<60 years old) patients when administered MSC therapy for chronic ischemic cardiomyopathy [89]. This is of great significance as the majority of the population with heart disease in need of cell-based therapy is comprised of aged individuals.

There is conflicting evidence regarding the potential of MSC therapy to promote carcinogenesis [90–93]. Whether the MSCs act as cancer cells themselves by undergoing spontaneous malignant transformation or they interact with surrounding tumor stromal elements remains unclear [94]. Rosland et al. [91] demonstrated spontaneous malignant transformation of human bone marrow-derived MSCs grown in long-term cultures. These cells proliferated more rapidly, were unable to undergo complete differentiation, and exhibited an altered morphology and phenotype compared to normal human MSCs. Additionally, when these transformed cells were injected into immunodeficient mice, histologic examination revealed rapid-growing tumor deposits found throughout the lung tissue. In contrast, in a study by Bernardo et al. [92], isolated human bone marrow-derived MSCs were grown in culture until they reached senescence or passage 25. Subsequently, cells were assessed genetically at different time points and various tumor-related proteins were measured. The majority of MSCs displayed a progressive decrease in proliferative capacity with shortened telomeres until reaching senescence. Importantly, cultured MSCs did not express telomerase activity or human telomerase reverse transcriptase transcripts and no chromosomal abnormalities or alternative lengthening of telomeres were noted. These data lend support to the safety of *ex vivo* MSC expansion and use in regenerative cell therapy. Nevertheless, careful attention to the functional, phenotypic, and genetic characterization of culture-expanded MSCs as well as other types of stem cells should still be given [94].

Sex differences exist in many disease states and particularly in cardiovascular disease [95, 96]. Post-menopausal women are at a higher risk of coronary artery disease, myocardial infarction, and atherosclerosis compared to pre-menopausal women and age matched men. Based on these findings, disparities in cardiovascular disease outcomes between women and men have been attributed to differences in sex steroid expression, predominantly estrogen. Sex differences also exist with respect to the roles of stem cells in organ repair and regeneration after injury. Female MSCs exhibit decreased apoptosis, decreased interleukin-6, decreased tumor necrosis factor, increased endothelial growth factor, and increased vascular endothelial growth factor expression compared to male donor MSCs [97]. Moreover, in a mouse myocardial infarction model, treatment with female MSCs produced greater recovery of cardiac functional parameters compared to male MSC treatment [98]. The effect of estradiol on MSCs contributes to these differences [99]. Understanding how stem cells are influenced by donor sex and recipient hormonal environment may help account for sex-related disparities in clinical outcomes as well as utilize the beneficial effects of these hormones to optimize transplanted stem cell function and survival.

3.3. Autologous versus allogeneic cell therapy.

An important issue in this new field is whether stem cells can be used as an allograft [2, 18, 28]. One potential advantage of allogeneic stem cells is their potential use as an "off-the-shelf" therapeutic agent, avoiding the need for bone marrow aspiration or cardiac biopsy and tissue culture delays prior to treatment. In addition, the function of autologous stem cells may be impaired in patients with comorbidities and/or advanced age, as described in the previous section [78, 79, 81, 84]. Regarding the most studied cell type, MSCs, the absence of major histocompatibility class (MHC) II antigens [100–102] and the secretion of T helper type 2 (TH2) cytokines characterize MSCs as immunoprivileged and immunosuppressive [102, 103], although there is some evidence that allogeneic MSCs may be cleared to a greater extent than autologous cell preparations possibly via formation of alloreactive antibodies [104]. Indeed, a meta-analysis of 82 preclinical studies [105] demonstrated that allogeneic therapy is equally as safe and effective as autologous therapy with MSCs, further suggesting that allogeneic MSCs are characteristically immunomodulatory.

The safety and therapeutic benefit of intravenous administration of allogeneic MSCs versus placebo has been demonstrated in patients after acute myocardial infarction [6, 106, 107]. Moreover, our group conducted phase I/II clinical trials comparing allogeneic and autologous MSCs delivered by transendocardial stem cell injection into patients with chronic ischemic cardiomyopathy and non-ischemic, dilated cardiomyopathy and showed that both MSC types are safe and clinically effective [2, 18, 29, 108]. These studies are paving the way for the development of allogeneic cell-based regenerative therapies for structural and functional disorders of the myocardium as well as other organs and disease processes [19, 20].

Other stem cell types may have similar immunologic properties. Regarding cardiac-derived stem cells, it has been reported that human CSCs may have immunomodulatory capacity in vitro [109], resembling the properties described for MSCs. A recent preclinical study using a porcine model of ischemic cardiomyopathy showed safety and efficacy of allogeneic CSCs alone and in combination with MSCs [110]. These preclinical findings require testing in future clinical trials. In this regard, the "ALLogeneic heart STem cells to Achieve myocardial Regeneration" (ALLSTAR; NCT01458405) clinical trial is investigating the safety and efficacy of allogeneic cardiospheres [48], in the absence of immunosuppression, after reporting positive preclinical findings [111, 112]. It is important to note that emerging evidence supports the idea that cardiospheres share the immunomodulatory properties of MSCs, since they express the classic markers, including CD105, CD90, and CD73 [113–115], and as such may be cardiac-specific stromal or mesenchymal cells. If these cardiac-derived $CD105^+$ cells are successfully used as an allograft, it would further support the notion that allogeneic cell therapy may be broadly applicable.

3.4. Selection of dose and delivery

As with any traditional new drug, establishing the optimal dose and delivery method is a critical part of the development of new stem cell therapies [36, 37, 116]. In a phase II-a study, drug development normally comprises an estimate of a non-effective dose and the highest tolerated dose, whereas in a phase II-b the objective is to determine the dose–response relationship by testing doses ranging from clinically non-effective to the highest tolerated. This paradigm is problematic in stem cell therapy development. Unlike traditional pharmacology, where pharmacokinetic and pharmacodynamics principles and methods are effectual, different principles and assumptions underlie the assessment of the correct dosing regimens in the field of stem cell therapy [36]. Stem cell therapies tested in phase I/II studies are not usually titrated to any specific pharmacodynamic effect targeting a particular physiological marker or pathway, although secondary assessments of dose on various biomarkers and/or cardiac functional parameters are done. The total number of cells administered is not necessarily proportional to the clinical effect, at least using the traditional clinical parameters, such as cardiac structure, functional capacity, and quality of life measurements. Indeed, the small number of preclinical [117–120] and clinical studies [2, 29, 121–125] that have examined cell dose have so far demonstrated conflicting results regarding the relationship between the quantity of cells delivered and clinical efficacy. The variability in cell types and delivery methods as well as the heterogeneous within and between-patient pathophysiology of cardiovascular disease contribute, at least in part, to the challenges in cell dose optimization [36, 116]. Thus, there is a need to design studies that compare both cell dose and delivery methods to determine which combination provides the best clinical outcome in a particular disease state (e.g., acute myocardial infarction vs. chronic heart failure). Other important factors that should be addressed in the field include the need to standardize the growing variety of stem cell sources (e.g. bone marrow, adipose tissue, placenta, umbilical cord, heart, etc.) and production methods and develop adequate methods for measuring the quality, potency, and/or biologic activity of stem cell preparations. This includes investigating concentration-dependent stem cell aggregation or clumping [126], which impacts cell viability and homing or engraftment in injured tissue, effects of culture media used for therapeutic stem cell preparation on tissue receptors or effector sites [127, 128], and effects of needle bore-induced shear forces on stem cell integrity [129, 130]. Moreover, given that the injected cells must survive and interact with the surrounding tissue microenvironment, the disease state must be consistent in order to compare cell dosing and clinical efficacy. Investigators planning to initiate clinical trials of stem cell therapy using a particular cell type and delivery method in a particular disease state should be mindful of any assumptions being made based on studies of other cell types and/or delivery methods and disease states and ensure that adequate attention has been paid to all of these as of yet incompletely understood variables.

3.5. Safety

Assessment of safety in phase I/II trials of stem cell therapy for cardiovascular disease is currently targeted to detect major concerns, including severe end-organ damage, such as myocardial infarction, stroke, or lung injury, severe allergic reactions, laboratory abnormalities, hemodynamic instability, or death. However, it is important to note that, as with all drugs and therapeutic agents, clinical safety can only be assessed with adequately powered long-term studies. This concern is particularly relevant with the cardiovascular end points usually assessed, such as functional capacity and quality of life. Although small phase I/II studies are useful to demonstrate improvement in these patient-centered outcomes, they may miss important safety signals and thus provide limited overall safety information.

3.6. Efficacy

Phase II trials are intentionally designed with a small number of patients and relatively short duration of follow up, and therefore do not have the power to assess the effect of the therapeutic agent on clinical outcomes such as mortality or hospitalization risk. The efficacy outcomes used in phase II trials are usually surrogate end points and translation biomarkers that correlate with mortality and/or hospitalization risk and can be assessed in the period of time of the trial. Therefore, the rationale for phase II clinical trials is to identify the potential clinical benefits of the novel therapy being tested, with minimal regard to statistical significance, on which phase III trials can then be based to confirm the findings in a larger population over a longer period of time.

The surrogate end points and translational biomarkers used for efficacy assessment in cell therapy phase II trials for cardiovascular disease create several challenges when designing phase III trials, which measure mortality or other clinical outcomes such as cardiac function. In other words, the efficacy end points in cell therapy phase II and phase III trials of cardiovascular disease are usually different. This uncertainty around the translatability and predictive value of changes in the phase II surrogate end point or biomarker to future changes in phase III clinical outcomes is a major issue for researchers and sponsors. There is evidence suggesting that although a potential surrogate marker or biomarker may have a strong association with clinical outcomes, it does not necessarily translate into a strong correlation with clinical outcomes in a phase III trial setting even if a favorable trend was observed in previous studies. For instance, improvement in left ventricular remodeling correlates significantly with

http://dx.doi.org/10.5772/intechopen.72949

clinical outcomes, such as mortality, in patients with heart failure. However, whereas some therapeutic agents that improve left ventricular remodeling also reduce mortality, other agents shown to reduce mortality have not been found to improve remodeling. Therefore, multiple surrogate endpoints and biomarkers are usually assessed in phase II trials in order to identify any signs of potential clinical efficacy.

4. Recommendations for the Design of Phase I/II trials of stem cell therapy for CVD

4.1. Identifying novel markers of clinical improvement

The development of novel surrogate markers of clinical benefit is crucial for the design of successful clinical trials [116]. An important issue is the identification of markers for subpopulations of patients with cardiovascular diseases based on the pathophysiology and the mechanism of action of the therapeutic agent. Novel applications such as genomics, proteomics, and bioengineering applications and devices can be utilized in this regard and to develop targeted therapies.

4.2. Matching end point selection with mechanism of action

In order to more accurately and precisely determine clinical efficacy in a trial, surrogate markers and biomarkers must be mechanistically affected by the studied drug or biologic agent [116]. It is important to recognize that repairing or regenerating injured cardiovascular tissues is a complex task involving various mechanisms of action that will have a different impact on different end points. For example, the antifibrotic effects of MSCs lead to a reduction in infarct scar size whereas the pro-angiogenic effects lead to neovascularization and increased perfusion, both of which improve cardiac function and structure. Therefore, future clinical trials must connect biological pathways, drug mechanisms of action, and underlying pathophysiology to be successful in developing efficacious novel therapies [116].

4.3. Use of a combination of efficacy and surrogate marker endpoints

As stated previously, in a phase II clinical trial the measure for success should not be linked to the achievement of statistical significance for a small number of primary endpoints in an effort to reduce the likelihood of a false positive finding [37, 116, 131]. The metric of reaching statistical significance for clinical endpoints is the goal of phase III trials. In this regard, the current recommendations for Phase II studies [37, 116, 131] are that many primary endpoints should be assessed, with each prospectively declared and its findings reported; the goal being to identify novel clinical benefits of the new therapy. In order to properly design phase III trials, investigators need to know all of the endpoint results as set out in the phase II study protocol. Moreover, to assess the consistency of the findings, the phase II investigators should select efficacy endpoints from different categories [37]. In cell therapy studies for cardiovascular disease, the important categories to evaluate include, (a) cardiac structure and function, such as infarct size, ventricular sphericity, ejection fraction, ventricular volumes, measures of contractility and diastolic performance, (b) biomarkers, such as atrial and brain natriuretic proteins, cardiac enzymes, TNF-alpha, C-reactive protein, micro-RNAs, and transcriptomic-based biomarkers, (c) physical functional capacity, such as 6 minute walk distance, peak walking time, and maximal oxygen consumption, and (d) quality of life, such as Minnesota Living with Heart Failure questionnaire, the Short Form-36, need for revascularization and recurrent myocardial infarction or heart failure exacerbations [37].

4.4. Development of novel analytical methods and guiding principles

The use of a combination of endpoints representing various different categories is expected to improve the development of cell-based therapies, but new analytical methods many need to be developed to manage these large quantities of data [37, 116, 131]. The data from the various categories needs to be evaluated using statistical methods that can generate a cumulative assessment of the impact of the intervention. The analytical methods utilized will need to be adapted based on the directionality and stratification of data, the disease process or clinical setting, specific patient population, and any potential discordant information that arises. These methods may help provide the power needed to detect differences in efficacy endpoints in phase II studies. However, as discussed previously, power is not as important as understanding the multitude of data points to avoid not translating a clinical benefit observed in a phase II study into a phase III trial. This approach highlights the importance of proper endpoint selection and consideration of individual components and decision-making guidelines.

Certain guiding principles for the assessment of phase II studies of cell-based therapies have been recommended [37]. These include "strength of association," "consistency and concordance," "coherence," "dose response," and "safety." Strength of association refers to whether the cell therapy being evaluated provides a greater clinical benefit than the control group. If the cell therapy has been beneficial compared to control in other studies involving different patient populations and/or clinical protocols, thus showing consistency and concordance, this benefit would support causality. In contrast, any differences in results between studies would need to be evaluated for possible biological reasons, such as differences in stem cell dose, manufacturing, delivery method, etc. Coherence is also an important principle as it links the observed clinical endpoints with the underlying physiologic effects of the cell-based therapy. For example, a therapy that improves cardiac structure and/or function and improves physical functioning or quality of life provides coherence to the results. Finally, the importance of dose response, sustainability of effect, and safety for cell-based therapies is similar to that of any pharmacologic drug, although there are unique aspects of cell-based therapies as discussed in the previous sections.

5. Need for regenerative medicine training programs and patient education

The number of academic and private physicians practicing regenerative medicine as well as the number of patients and chronic conditions being treated with cell-based therapies has grown exponentially in the past decade [132–136]. Although clinical trials throughout the world have been or are being conducted and reported through clinicaltrials.gov, and governmental regulatory bodies provide some oversight [134, 137, 138], there is a growing concern that physicians without prior or proper training in cell-based therapeutics are treating patients with stem cells from various sources with little or no evidence of safety or efficacy [132, 133, 136, 139]. To add to these concerns, there is a growing demand to deregulate the use of these therapies [140–144]. The rules of the FDA as well as the European Medicines Agency define stem cells modified outside the body as medicines and therefore under their regulatory oversight [134, 137, 138]. However, commercial promotion of unsupported therapeutic uses of stem cells has become a world-wide problem that has proven resistant to regulatory efforts and has created unsafe situations that have resulted in harm to patients, both physically and psychologically (i.e., false promises of cure), and avoidable, punitive conflicts between governmental regulatory agencies and physicians [132–135, 137–140, 143, 145, 146]. One approach that has been proposed to promote compliance and uniformity in this growing field is the implementation of physician training programs at academic institutions [135].

It is imperative that the global biomedical research community be the leaders in developing educational programs to not only train physicians, but also inform patients, the general public, and governmental agencies on the appropriate development, investigation, and clinical use of cell-based therapies [37, 132, 147, 148]. It was with this goal in mind that the National Institutes of Health-sponsored cardiovascular cell therapy network (CCTRN) supports physician training programs that provide expertise in all aspects of regenerative medicine. The mission of the CCTRN is to "achieve public health advances for the treatment of cardiovascular diseases, through the conduct and dissemination of collaborative research leading to evidence-based treatment options and improved outcome for patients with heart disease" (https://sph.uth.edu/research/centers/ccct/cctrn/about-us.htm) [37, 147, 148].

Author details

Ivonne H. Schulman[1,2]*, Wayne Balkan[1], Russell Saltzman[1], Daniel DaFonseca[1], Lina V. Caceres[1], Cindy Delgado[1], Marietsy V. Pujol[1], Kevin N. Ramdas[1], Jairo Tovar[1], Mayra Vidro-Casiano[1] and Joshua M. Hare[1]

*Address all correspondence to: ischulman@med.miami.edu

1 The Interdisciplinary Stem Cell Institute, University of Miami Miller School of Medicine, Miami, Florida, U.S.A.

2 Katz Family Division of Nephrology, University of Miami Miller School of Medicine, Miami, Florida, U.S.A.

References

[1] Heldman AW, DiFede DL, Fishman JE, et al. Transendocardial mesenchymal stem cells and mononuclear bone marrow cells for ischemic cardiomyopathy: The TAC-HFT randomized trial. Journal of the American Medical Association. 2014 Jan 1;**311**(1):62-73. DOI: 10.1001/jama.2013.282909

[2] Hare JM, Fishman JE, Gerstenblith G, et al. Comparison of allogeneic vs autologous bone marrow-derived mesenchymal stem cells delivered by transendocardial injection in patients with ischemic cardiomyopathy: The POSEIDON randomized trial. Journal of the American Medical Association. 2012 Dec 12;**308**(22):2369-2379. DOI: 10.1001/jama.2012.25321

[3] Le Blanc K, Frassoni F, Ball L, et al. Mesenchymal stem cells for treatment of steroid-resistant, severe, acute graft-versus-host disease: A phase II study. Lancet. 2008 May 10;**371**(9624):1579-1586. DOI: 10.1016/S0140-6736(08)60690-X

[4] Le Blanc K, Rasmusson I, Sundberg B, et al. Treatment of severe acute graft-versus-host disease with third party haploidentical mesenchymal stem cells. Lancet. 2004 May 1;**363** (9419):1439-1441. DOI: 10.1016/S0140-6736(04)16104-7

[5] Liang J, Zhang H, Hua B, et al. Allogenic mesenchymal stem cells transplantation in refractory systemic lupus erythematosus: A pilot clinical study. Annals of the Rheumatic Diseases. 2010 Aug;**69**(8):1423-1429. DOI: 10.1136/ard.2009.123463

[6] Hare JM, Traverse JH, Henry TD, et al. A randomized, double-blind, placebo-controlled, dose-escalation study of intravenous adult human mesenchymal stem cells (prochymal) after acute myocardial infarction. Journal of the American College of Cardiology. 2009 Dec 8;**54**(24):2277-2286. DOI: 10.1016/j.jacc.2009.06.055

[7] Weiss DJ, Casaburi R, Flannery R, et al. A placebo-controlled randomized trial of mesenchymal stem cells in chronic obstructive pulmonary disease. Chest. 2012 Nov 22;**143**(6):1590-1598 DOI: 10.1378/chest.12-2094

[8] Lalu MM, McIntyre L, Pugliese C, et al. Safety of cell therapy with mesenchymal stromal cells (SafeCell): A systematic review and meta-analysis of clinical trials. PLoS One. 2012;**7**(10):e47559. DOI: 10.1371/journal.pone.0047559

[9] Tan J, Wu W, Xu X, et al. Induction therapy with autologous mesenchymal stem cells in living-related kidney transplants: A randomized controlled trial. JAMA : The Journal of the American Medical Association. 2012 Mar 21;**307**(11):1169-1177. DOI: 10.1001/jama.2012.316

[10] Karussis D, Karageorgiou C, Vaknin-Dembinsky A, et al. Safety and immunological effects of mesenchymal stem cell transplantation in patients with multiple sclerosis and amyotrophic lateral sclerosis. Archives of Neurology. 2010 Oct;**67**(10):1187-1194. DOI: 10.1001/archneurol.2010.248

[11] Mazzini L, Ferrero I, Luparello V, et al. Mesenchymal stem cell transplantation in amyotrophic lateral sclerosis: A phase I clinical trial. Experimental Neurology. 2010 May;**223**(1):229-237. DOI: 10.1016/j.expneurol.2009.08.007

[12] Peng L, Xie DY, Lin BL, et al. Autologous bone marrow mesenchymal stem cell transplantation in liver failure patients caused by hepatitis B: Short-term and long-term outcomes. Hepatology. 2011 Sep 2;**54**(3):820-828. DOI: 10.1002/hep.24434

[13] Kharaziha P, Hellstrom PM, Noorinayer B, et al. Improvement of liver function in liver cirrhosis patients after autologous mesenchymal stem cell injection: A phase I-II clinical trial. European Journal of Gastroenterology & Hepatology. 2009 Oct;**21**(10):1199-1205. DOI: 10.1097/MEG.0b013e32832a1f6c

[14] Honmou O, Houkin K, Matsunaga T, et al. Intravenous administration of auto serum-expanded autologous mesenchymal stem cells in stroke. Brain: A Journal of Neurology. 2011 Jun;**134**(Pt 6):1790-1807. DOI: 10.1093/brain/awr063

[15] Lee JS, Hong JM, Moon GJ, et al. A long-term follow-up study of intravenous autologous mesenchymal stem cell transplantation in patients with ischemic stroke. Stem Cells. 2010 Jun;**28**(6):1099-1106. DOI: 10.1002/stem.430

[16] Lee PH, Lee JE, Kim HS, et al. A randomized trial of mesenchymal stem cells in multiple system atrophy. Annals of Neurology. 2012 Jul;**72**(1):32-40. DOI: 10.1002/ana.23612

[17] Badiavas AR, Badiavas EV. Potential benefits of allogeneic bone marrow mesenchymal stem cells for wound healing. Expert Opinion on Biological Therapy. 2011 Nov;**11**(11): 1447-1454. DOI: 10.1517/14712598.2011.606212

[18] Hare JM, DiFede DL, Rieger AC, et al. Randomized comparison of allogeneic versus autologous mesenchymal stem cells for nonischemic dilated cardiomyopathy: POSEIDON-DCM trial. Journal of the American College of Cardiology. 2017 Feb 07;**69**(5):526-537. DOI: 10.1016/j.jacc.2016.11.009

[19] Golpanian S, DiFede DL, Khan A, et al. Allogeneic human mesenchymal stem cell infusions for aging frailty. The Journals of Gerontology Series A, Biological Sciences and Medical Sciences. 2017 Apr 21;**72**(11):1505-1512. DOI: 10.1093/gerona/glx056

[20] Glassberg MK, Minkiewicz J, Toonkel RL, et al. Allogeneic human mesenchymal stem cells in patients with idiopathic pulmonary fibrosis via intravenous delivery (AETHER): A phase I safety clinical trial. Chest. 2017 May;**151**(5):971-981. DOI: 10.1016/j.chest.2016.10.061

[21] Hatzistergos KE, Quevedo H, Oskouei BN, et al. Bone marrow mesenchymal stem cells stimulate cardiac stem cell proliferation and differentiation. Circulation Research. 2010 Oct 1;**107**(7):913-922. DOI: 10.1161/CIRCRESAHA.110.222703

[22] Quevedo HC, Hatzistergos KE, Oskouei BN, et al. Allogeneic mesenchymal stem cells restore cardiac function in chronic ischemic cardiomyopathy via trilineage differentiating capacity. Proceedings of the National Academy of Sciences of the United States of America. 2009 Aug 18;**106**(33):14022-14027. DOI: 10.1073/pnas.0903201106

[23] Schuleri KH, Feigenbaum GS, Centola M, et al. Autologous mesenchymal stem cells produce reverse remodelling in chronic ischaemic cardiomyopathy. European Heart Journal. 2009 Nov;**30**(22):2722-2732. DOI: 10.1093/eurheartj/ehp265

[24] Williams AR, Hatzistergos KE, Addicott B, et al. Enhanced effect of combining human cardiac stem cells and bone marrow mesenchymal stem cells to reduce infarct size and

to restore cardiac function after myocardial infarction. Circulation. 2013;**127**(2):213-223. DOI: 10.1161/circulationaha.112.131110

[25] Karantalis V, Suncion-Loescher VY, Bagno L, et al. Synergistic effects of combined cell therapy for chronic ischemic cardiomyopathy. Journal of the American College of Cardiology. 2015 Nov 3;**66**(18):1990-1999. DOI: 10.1016/j.jacc.2015.08.879

[26] Kulandavelu S, Karantalis V, Fritsch J, et al. Pim1 kinase overexpression enhances ckit+ cardiac stem cell cardiac repair following myocardial infarction in swine. Journal of the American College of Cardiology. 2016 Dec 06;**68**(22):2454-2464. DOI: 10.1016/j.jacc.2016.09.925

[27] Kanelidis AJ, Premer C, Lopez J, et al. Route of delivery modulates the efficacy of mesenchymal stem cell therapy for myocardial infarction: A meta-analysis of preclinical studies and clinical trials. Circulation Research. 2017 Mar 31;**120**(7):1139-1150. DOI: 10.1161/CIRCRESAHA.116.309819

[28] Karantalis V, Schulman IH, Balkan W, et al. Allogeneic cell therapy: A new paradigm in therapeutics. Circulation Research. 2015 Jan 2;**116**(1):12-15. DOI: 10.1161/CIRCRESAHA.114.305495

[29] Florea V, Rieger AC, Difede DL, et al. Dose comparison study of allogeneic mesenchymal stem cells in patients with ischemic cardiomyopathy (the TRIDENT study). Circulation Research. 2017 Sep 18. DOI: 10.1161/CIRCRESAHA.117.311827

[30] Khan AR, Farid TA, Pathan A, et al. Impact of cell therapy on myocardial perfusion and cardiovascular outcomes in patients with angina refractory to medical therapy: A systematic review and meta-analysis. Circulation Research. 2016 Mar 18;**118**(6):984-993. DOI: 10.1161/CIRCRESAHA.115.308056

[31] Florea V, Balkan W, Schulman IH, et al. Cell therapy augments myocardial perfusion and improves quality of life in patients with refractory angina. Circulation Research. 2016 Mar 18;**118**(6):911-915. DOI: 10.1161/CIRCRESAHA.116.308409

[32] Bolli R, Chugh AR, D'Amario D, et al. Cardiac stem cells in patients with ischaemic cardiomyopathy (SCIPIO): Initial results of a randomised phase 1 trial. Lancet. 2011 Nov 26;**378**(9806):1847-1857. DOI: 10.1016/S0140-6736(11)61590-0

[33] Bolli RCA, D'Amario D, Stoddard MF, Ikram S, Wagner SG, Beache GM, Leri A, Hosoda T, Loughran JH, et al. Use of cardiac stem cells for the treatment of heart failure: Translation from the bench to the clinical setting. Circulation Research. 2010;**107**:e33

[34] Makkar RR, Smith RR, Cheng K, et al. Intracoronary cardiosphere-derived cells for heart regeneration after myocardial infarction (CADUCEUS): A prospective, randomised phase 1 trial. Lancet. 2012 Mar 10;**379**(9819):895-904. DOI: 10.1016/S0140-6736(12)60195-0

[35] Karantalis V, Hare JM. Use of mesenchymal stem cells for therapy of cardiac disease. Circulation Research. 2015 Apr 10;**116**(8):1413-1430. DOI: 10.1161/CIRCRESAHA.116.303614

[36] Golpanian S, Schulman IH, Ebert RF, et al. Concise review: Review and perspective of cell dosage and routes of administration from preclinical and clinical studies of stem cell

therapy for heart disease. Stem Cells Translational Medicine. 2016 Feb;**5**(2):186-191. DOI: 10.5966/sctm.2015-0101

[37] Hare JM, Bolli R, Cooke JP, et al. Phase II clinical research design in cardiology: Learning the right lessons too well: Observations and recommendations from the cardiovascular cell therapy research network (CCTRN). Circulation. 2013 Apr 16;**127**(15):1630-1635. DOI: 10.1161/CIRCULATIONAHA.112.000779

[38] Golpanian S, Wolf A, Hatzistergos KE, et al. Rebuilding the damaged heart: Mesenchymal stem cells, cell-based therapy, and engineered heart tissue. Physiological Reviews. 2016 Jul;**96**(3):1127-1168. DOI: 10.1152/physrev.00019.2015

[39] Hatzistergos KE, Saur D, Seidler B, et al. Stimulatory effects of mesenchymal stem cells on cKit+ cardiac stem cells are mediated by SDF1/CXCR4 and SCF/cKit signaling pathways. Circulation Research. 2016 Sep 30;**119**(8):921-930. DOI: 10.1161/CIRCRESAHA.116.309281

[40] Premer C, Blum A, Bellio MA, et al. Allogeneic mesenchymal stem cells restore endothelial function in heart failure by stimulating endothelial progenitor cells. eBioMedicine. 2015;**2**(5):467-475. DOI: 10.1016/j.ebiom.2015.03.020

[41] Kepplinger EE. FDA's expedited approval mechanisms for new drug products. Biotechnology Law Report. 2015;**34**(1):15-37. DOI: 10.1089/blr.2015.9999

[42] Darrow JJ, Avorn J, Kesselheim AS. New FDA breakthrough-drug category — Implications for patients. The New England Journal of Medicine. 2014;**370**(13):1252-1258. DOI: 10.1056/NEJMhle1311493

[43] Newton PNSD, Ashley EA, Ravinetto R, Green MD, Kuile FO, et al. Quality assurance of drugs used in clinical trials: Proposal for adapting guidelines. BMJ: British Medical Journal (Online). 2015;**350**:h602. DOI: 10.1136/bmj.h602

[44] Pittenger MF, Mackay AM, Beck SC, et al. Multilineage potential of adult human mesenchymal stem cells. Science. 1999 Apr 2;**284**(5411):143-147

[45] Williams AR, Hare JM. Mesenchymal stem cells: Biology, pathophysiology, translational findings, and therapeutic implications for cardiac disease. Circulation Research. 2011 Sep 30;**109**(8):923-940. DOI: 10.1161/CIRCRESAHA.111.243147

[46] von Bahr L, Batsis I, Moll G, et al. Analysis of tissues following mesenchymal stromal cell therapy in humans indicates limited long-term engraftment and no ectopic tissue formation. Stem Cells. 2012 Jul;**30**(7):1575-1578. DOI: 10.1002/stem.1118

[47] Messina E, De Angelis L, Frati G, et al. Isolation and expansion of adult cardiac stem cells from human and murine heart. Circulation Research. 2004 Oct 29;**95**(9):911-921. DOI: 10.1161/01.RES.0000147315.71699.51

[48] Smith RR, Barile L, Cho HC, et al. Regenerative potential of cardiosphere-derived cells expanded from percutaneous endomyocardial biopsy specimens. Circulation. 2007 Feb 20;**115**(7):896-908. DOI: 10.1161/CIRCULATIONAHA.106.655209

[49] Beltrami AP, Barlucchi L, Torella D, et al. Adult cardiac stem cells are multipotent and support myocardial regeneration. Cell. 2003 Sep 19;**114**(6):763-776. DOI: S009286740300 6871 [pii]

[50] Urbanek K, Torella D, Sheikh F, et al. Myocardial regeneration by activation of multipotent cardiac stem cells in ischemic heart failure. Proceedings of the National Academy of Sciences of the United States of America. 2005 Jun 14;**102**(24):8692-8697. DOI: 10.1073/pnas.0500169102

[51] Rodrigues CO, Shehadeh LA, Hoosien M, et al. Heterogeneity in SDF-1 expression defines the vasculogenic potential of adult cardiac progenitor cells. PLoS One. 2011;**6** (8):e24013. DOI: 10.1371/journal.pone.0024013

[52] Hatzistergos KE, Takeuchi LM, Saur D, et al. cKit+ cardiac progenitors of neural crest origin. Proceedings of the National Academy of Sciences of the United States of America. 2015 Oct 20;**112**(42):13051-13056. DOI: 10.1073/pnas.1517201112

[53] van Berlo JH, Kanisicak O, Maillet M, et al. c-kit+ cells minimally contribute cardiomyocytes to the heart. Nature. 2014 May 15;**509**(7500):337-341. DOI: 10.1038/nature13309

[54] Hatzistergos KE, Hare JM. Murine models demonstrate distinct vasculogenic and cardiomyogenic cKit+ lineages in the heart. Circulation Research. 2016 Feb 5;**118**(3):382-387. DOI: 10.1161/CIRCRESAHA.115.308061

[55] Eschenhagen T, Bolli R, Braun T, et al. Cardiomyocyte regeneration: A consensus statement. Circulation. 2017 Aug 15;**136**(7):680-686. DOI: 10.1161/CIRCULATIONAHA.117.029343

[56] Zwetsloot PP, Vegh AM, OLSJ J, et al. Cardiac stem cell treatment in myocardial infarction: A systematic review and meta-analysis of preclinical studies. Circulation Research. 2016 Apr 15;**118**(8):1223-1232. DOI: 10.1161/CIRCRESAHA.115.307676

[57] Bearzi C, Rota M, Hosoda T, et al. Human cardiac stem cells. Proceedings of the National Academy of Sciences of the United States of America. 2007 Aug 28;**104** (35):14068-14073. DOI: 10.1073/pnas.0706760104: 0706760104 [pii]

[58] Linke A, Muller P, Nurzynska D, et al. Stem cells in the dog heart are self-renewing, clonogenic, and multipotent and regenerate infarcted myocardium, improving cardiac function. Proceedings of the National Academy of Sciences of the United States of America. 2005 Jun 21;**102**(25):8966-8971. DOI: 10.1073/pnas.0502678102

[59] Rota M, Padin-Iruegas ME, Misao Y, et al. Local activation or implantation of cardiac progenitor cells rescues scarred infarcted myocardium improving cardiac function. Circulation Research. 2008 Jul 3;**103**(1):107-116. DOI: 10.1161/CIRCRESAHA.108.178525

[60] Chugh AR, Beache GM, Loughran JH, et al. Administration of cardiac stem cells in patients with ischemic cardiomyopathy: The SCIPIO trial: Surgical aspects and interim analysis of myocardial function and viability by magnetic resonance. Circulation. 2012 Sep 11;**126**(11 Suppl 1):S54-S64. DOI: 10.1161/CIRCULATIONAHA.112.092627

[61] Bolli R, Chugh AR, D'Amario D, Loughran JH, Stoddard MF, Ikram S, Wagner SG, Beache GM, Leri A, Hosoda T, Goihberg P, Fiorini C, Solankhi N, Fahsah I, Elmore JB, Rokosh DG, Slaughter MS, Kajstura J, Anversa P. Effect of cardiac stem cells in patients with ischemic cardiomyopathy: Interim results of the SCIPIO trial up to 2 years after therapy. Circulation. 2012;**126**(23):2784

[62] Takehara N et al. The ALCADIA (autologous human cardiac-derived stem cell to treat ischemic cardiomyopathy). Trial. 2012;**126**:2776-2799

[63] Lee ST, White AJ, Matsushita S, et al. Intramyocardial injection of autologous cardiospheres or cardiosphere-derived cells preserves function and minimizes adverse ventricular remodeling in pigs with heart failure post-myocardial infarction. Journal of the American College of Cardiology. 2011 Jan 25;**57**(4):455-465. DOI: 10.1016/j.jacc.2010.07.049

[64] Erbs S, Linke A, Schachinger V, et al. Restoration of microvascular function in the infarct-related artery by intracoronary transplantation of bone marrow progenitor cells in patients with acute myocardial infarction: The Doppler substudy of the reinfusion of enriched progenitor cells and infarct remodeling in acute myocardial infarction (REPAIR-AMI) trial. Circulation. 2007 Jul 24;**116**(4):366-374. DOI: 10.1161/CIRCULATIONAHA.106.671545

[65] Schachinger V, Erbs S, Elsasser A, et al. Improved clinical outcome after intracoronary administration of bone-marrow-derived progenitor cells in acute myocardial infarction: Final 1-year results of the REPAIR-AMI trial. European Heart Journal. 2006 Dec;**27**(23): 2775-2783. DOI: 10.1093/eurheartj/ehl388

[66] Surder D, Schwitter J, Moccetti T, et al. Cell-based therapy for myocardial repair in patients with acute myocardial infarction: Rationale and study design of the SWiss multicenter intracoronary stem cells study in acute myocardial infarction (SWISS-AMI). American Heart Journal. 2010 Jul;**160**(1):58-64. DOI: 10.1016/j.ahj.2010.03.039

[67] Traverse JH, Henry TD, Ellis SG, et al. Effect of intracoronary delivery of autologous bone marrow mononuclear cells 2 to 3 weeks following acute myocardial infarction on left ventricular function: The LateTIME randomized trial. JAMA. 2011 Nov 16;**306**(19): 2110-2119. DOI: 10.1001/jama.2011.1670

[68] Traverse JH, Henry TD, Pepine CJ, et al. Effect of the use and timing of bone marrow mononuclear cell delivery on left ventricular function after acute myocardial infarction: The TIME randomized trial. JAMA. 2012 Nov;**6**:1-10. DOI: 10.1001/jama.2012.28726

[69] Surder D, Manka R, Moccetti T, Rufibach K, Astori G, Lo Cicero V, Soncin S, Turchetto L, Radrizzani M, Windecker S, Moschovitis A, Wahl A, Erne P, Auf der Maur C, Soldati G, Buhler I, Wyss C, Schwitter J, Landmesser U, Lusher TF, Corti R. Results of the Swiss multicenter intracoronary stem cells study in acute myocardial infarction (Swiss Ami) trial. Circulation. 2012;**126**(23):2783

[70] Perin EC, Willerson JT, Pepine CJ, et al. Effect of transendocardial delivery of autologous bone marrow mononuclear cells on functional capacity, left ventricular function, and perfusion in chronic heart failure: The FOCUS-CCTRN trial. Journal of the American Medical Association. 2012 Apr 25;**307**(16):1717-1726. DOI: 10.1001/jama.2012.418

[71] Cogle CR, Wise E, Meacham AM, et al. Detailed analysis of bone marrow from patients with ischemic heart disease and left ventricular dysfunction: BM CD34, CD11b, and clonogenic capacity as biomarkers for clinical outcomes. Circulation Research. 2014 Oct 24;**115**(10):867-874. DOI: 10.1161/CIRCRESAHA.115.304353

[72] Kim MC, Kini A, Sharma SK. Refractory angina pectoris: Mechanism and therapeutic options. Journal of the American College of Cardiology. 2002 Mar 20;**39**(6):923-934

[73] Khan AR, Farid TA, Pathan A, et al. Impact of cell therapy on myocardial perfusion and cardiovascular outcomes in patients with angina refractory to medical therapy: A systematic review and meta-analysis. Circulation Research. 2016 Jan 13. DOI: 10.1161/CIRCRESAHA.115.308056

[74] Li N, Yang YJ, Zhang Q, et al. Stem cell therapy is a promising tool for refractory angina: A meta-analysis of randomized controlled trials. The Canadian Journal of Cardiology. 2013 Aug;**29**(8):908-914. DOI: 10.1016/j.cjca.2012.12.003

[75] Fisher SA, Doree C, Brunskill SJ, et al. Bone marrow stem cell treatment for ischemic heart disease in patients with no option of revascularization: A systematic review and meta-analysis. PLoS One. 2013;**8**(6):e64669. DOI: 10.1371/journal.pone.0064669

[76] Jeevanantham V, Butler M, Saad A, et al. Adult bone marrow cell therapy improves survival and induces long-term improvement in cardiac parameters: A systematic review and meta-analysis. Circulation. 2012 Jul 31;**126**(5):551-568. DOI: 10.1161/CIRCULATIONAHA.111.086074

[77] Clifford DM, Fisher SA, Brunskill SJ, et al. Stem cell treatment for acute myocardial infarction. Cochrane Database of Systematic Reviews. 2012;**2**:CD006536. DOI: 10.1002/14651858.CD006536.pub3

[78] KR Y, Kang KS. Aging-related genes in mesenchymal stem cells: A mini-review. Gerontology. 2013;**59**(6):557-563. DOI: 10.1159/000353857

[79] Raggi C, Berardi AC. Mesenchymal stem cells, aging and regenerative medicine. Muscles, Ligaments and Tendons Journal. 2012 Jul;**2**(3):239-242

[80] Zhuo Y, Li SH, Chen MS, et al. Aging impairs the angiogenic response to ischemic injury and the activity of implanted cells: Combined consequences for cell therapy in older recipients. The Journal of Thoracic and Cardiovascular Surgery. 2010 May;**139**(5):1286-1294, 94 e1-2). DOI: 10.1016/j.jtcvs.2009.08.052

[81] Jones DL, Rando TA. Emerging models and paradigms for stem cell ageing. Nature Cell Biology. 2011 May;**13**(5):506-512. DOI: 10.1038/ncb0511-506

[82] Sousa-Victor P, Gutarra S, Garcia-Prat L, et al. Geriatric muscle stem cells switch reversible quiescence into senescence. Nature. 2014 Feb 12. DOI: 10.1038/nature13013

[83] Geissler S, Textor M, Schmidt-Bleek K, et al. In serum veritas-in serum sanitas? Cell non-autonomous aging compromises differentiation and survival of mesenchymal stromal cells via the oxidative stress pathway. Cell Death & Disease. 2013;**4**:e970. DOI: 10.1038/cddis.2013.501

[84] Ballard VL. Stem cells for heart failure in the aging heart. Heart Failure Reviews. 2010 Sep;**15**(5):447-456. DOI: 10.1007/s10741-010-9160-z

[85] Li TS, Kubo M, Ueda K, et al. Impaired angiogenic potency of bone marrow cells from patients with advanced age, anemia, and renal failure. The Journal of Thoracic and Cardiovascular Surgery. 2010 Feb;**139**(2):459-465. DOI: 10.1016/j.jtcvs.2009.07.053

[86] Li TS, Kubo M, Ueda K, et al. Identification of risk factors related to poor angiogenic potency of bone marrow cells from different patients. Circulation. 2009 Sep 15;**120**(11 Suppl):S255-S261. DOI: 10.1161/CIRCULATIONAHA.108.837039

[87] Giannotti G, Doerries C, Mocharla PS, et al. Impaired endothelial repair capacity of early endothelial progenitor cells in prehypertension: Relation to endothelial dysfunction. Hypertension. 2010 Jun;**55**(6):1389-1397. DOI: 10.1161/HYPERTENSIONAHA.109.141614

[88] Kissel CK, Lehmann R, Assmus B, et al. Selective functional exhaustion of hematopoietic progenitor cells in the bone marrow of patients with postinfarction heart failure. Journal of the American College of Cardiology. 2007 Jun 19;**49**(24):2341-2349. DOI: 10.1016/j.jacc.2007.01.095

[89] Golpanian S, El-Khorazaty J, Mendizabal A, et al. Effect of aging on human mesenchymal stem cell therapy in ischemic cardiomyopathy patients. Journal of the American College of Cardiology. 2015 Jan 20;**65**(2):125-132. DOI: 10.1016/j.jacc.2014.10.040

[90] Li H, Fan X, Kovi RC, et al. Spontaneous expression of embryonic factors and p53 point mutations in aged mesenchymal stem cells: A model of age-related tumorigenesis in mice. Cancer Research. 2007 Nov 15;**67**(22):10889-10898. DOI: 10.1158/0008-5472.CAN-07-2665

[91] Rosland GV, Svendsen A, Torsvik A, et al. Long-term cultures of bone marrow-derived human mesenchymal stem cells frequently undergo spontaneous malignant transformation. Cancer Research. 2009 Jul 1;**69**(13):5331-5339. DOI: 10.1158/0008-5472.CAN-08-4630

[92] Bernardo ME, Zaffaroni N, Novara F, et al. Human bone marrow derived mesenchymal stem cells do not undergo transformation after long-term in vitro culture and do not exhibit telomere maintenance mechanisms. Cancer Research. 2007 Oct 1;**67**(19):9142-9149. DOI: 10.1158/0008-5472.CAN-06-4690

[93] Hatzistergos KE, Blum A, Ince T, et al. What is the oncologic risk of stem cell treatment for heart disease? Circulation Research. 2011 May 27;**108**(11):1300-1303. DOI: 10.1161/CIRCRESAHA.111.246611

[94] Tysnes BB, Bjerkvig R. Cancer initiation and progression: involvement of stem cells and the microenvironment. Biochimica et Biophysica Acta. 2007 Jun;**1775**(2):283-297. DOI: 10.1016/j.bbcan.2007.01.001

[95] Merz AA, Cheng S. Sex differences in cardiovascular ageing. Heart. 2016 Jun 01;**102**(11):825-831. DOI: 10.1136/heartjnl-2015-308769

[96] Cheng S, Xanthakis V, Sullivan LM, et al. Correlates of echocardiographic indices of cardiac remodeling over the adult life course: Longitudinal observations from the Framingham

heart study. Circulation. 2010 Aug 10;**122**(6):570-578. DOI: 10.1161/CIRCULATIONAHA.110.937821

[97] Crisostomo PR, Wang M, Herring CM, et al. Gender differences in injury induced mesenchymal stem cell apoptosis and VEGF, TNF, IL-6 expression: Role of the 55 kDa TNF receptor (TNFR1). Journal of Molecular and Cellular Cardiology. 2007 Jan;**42**(1):142-149. DOI: 10.1016/j.yjmcc.2006.09.016

[98] Crisostomo PR, Markel TA, Wang M, et al. In the adult mesenchymal stem cell population, source gender is a biologically relevant aspect of protective power. Surgery. 2007 Aug;**142**(2):215-221. DOI: 10.1016/j.surg.2007.04.013

[99] Herrmann JL, Abarbanell AM, Weil BR, et al. Gender dimorphisms in progenitor and stem cell function in cardiovascular disease. Journal of Cardiovascular Translational Research. 2010 Apr;**3**(2):103-113. DOI: 10.1007/s12265-009-9149-y

[100] Le Blanc K, Tammik C, Rosendahl K, et al. HLA expression and immunologic properties of differentiated and undifferentiated mesenchymal stem cells. Experimental Hematology. 2003 Oct;**31**(10):890-896

[101] Le Blanc K, Tammik L, Sundberg B, et al. Mesenchymal stem cells inhibit and stimulate mixed lymphocyte cultures and mitogenic responses independently of the major histocompatibility complex. Scandinavian Journal of Immunology. 2003 Jan;**57**(1):11-20

[102] Klyushnenkova E, Mosca JD, Zernetkina V, et al. T cell responses to allogeneic human mesenchymal stem cells: Immunogenicity, tolerance, and suppression. Journal of Biomedical Science. 2005;**12**(1):47-57. DOI: 10.1007/s11373-004-8183-7

[103] Beyth S, Borovsky Z, Mevorach D, et al. Human mesenchymal stem cells alter antigen-presenting cell maturation and induce T-cell unresponsiveness. Blood. 2005 Mar 1;**105**(5):2214-2219. DOI: 10.1182/blood-2004-07-2921

[104] Huang XP, Sun Z, Miyagi Y, et al. Differentiation of allogeneic mesenchymal stem cells induces immunogenicity and limits their long-term benefits for myocardial repair. Circulation. 2010 Dec 7;**122**(23):2419-2429. DOI: 10.1161/CIRCULATIONAHA.110.955971

[105] OLSJ J, Eding JE, Vesterinen HM, et al. Similar effect of autologous and allogeneic cell therapy for ischemic heart disease: Systematic review and meta-analysis of large animal studies. Circulation Research. 2015 Jan 2;**116**(1):80-86. DOI: 10.1161/circresaha.116.304872

[106] Chullikana A, Majumdar AS, Gottipamula S, et al. Randomized, double-blind, phase I/II study of intravenous allogeneic mesenchymal stromal cells in acute myocardial infarction. Cytotherapy. 2015 Mar;**17**(3):250-261. DOI: 10.1016/j.jcyt.2014.10.009

[107] Penn MS, Ellis S, Gandhi S, et al. Adventitial delivery of an allogeneic bone marrow-derived adherent stem cell in acute myocardial infarction: Phase I clinical study. Circulation Research. 2012 Jan 20;**110**(2):304-311. DOI: 10.1161/CIRCRESAHA.111.253427

[108] Suncion VY, Ghersin E, Fishman J, et al. Does transendocardial injection of mesenchymal stem cells improve myocardial function locally or globally? An analysis from the POSEIDON randomized trial. Circulation Research. 2014 Apr 11;**114**(8):1292-1301. DOI: 10.1161/CIRCRESAHA.114.302854

[109] Lauden L, Boukouaci W, Borlado LR, et al. Allogenicity of human cardiac stem/progenitor cells orchestrated by programmed death ligand 1. Circulation Research. 2013 Feb 1; **112**(3):451-464. DOI: 10.1161/CIRCRESAHA.112.276501

[110] Makoto Natsumeda VF, Castellanos AM, Tompkins BA, Landin AM, Fritsch J, Collon K, Vincent L, Kanelidis AJ, Rodriguez J, Rosado M, Schulman IH, Balkan W, Mitrani R, Hare J. The combination of allogeneic mesenchymal stem cells and cardiac stem cells produce synergistic effects in cardiac regeneration. Circulation. 2016;**134**(Suppl 1):A19681

[111] Tseliou E, Pollan S, Malliaras K, et al. Allogeneic cardiospheres safely boost cardiac function and attenuate adverse remodeling after myocardial infarction in immunologically mismatched rat strains. Journal of the American College of Cardiology. 2013 Mar 12;**61**(10):1108-1119. DOI: 10.1016/j.jacc.2012.10.052

[112] Malliaras K, Li TS, Luthringer D, et al. Safety and efficacy of allogeneic cell therapy in infarcted rats transplanted with mismatched cardiosphere-derived cells. Circulation. 2012 Jan 3;**125**(1):100-112. DOI: 10.1161/CIRCULATIONAHA.111.042598

[113] Tateishi K, Ashihara E, Honsho S, et al. Human cardiac stem cells exhibit mesenchymal features and are maintained through Akt/GSK-3beta signaling. Biochemical and Biophysical Research Communications. 2007 Jan 19;**352**(3):635-641. DOI: 10.1016/j.bbrc.2006.11.096

[114] Pouly J, Bruneval P, Mandet C, et al. Cardiac stem cells in the real world. The Journal of Thoracic and Cardiovascular Surgery. 2008 Mar;**135**(3):673-678. DOI: 10.1016/j.jtcvs.2007.10.024

[115] Mishra R, Vijayan K, Colletti EJ, et al. Characterization and functionality of cardiac progenitor cells in congenital heart patients. Circulation. 2011 Feb 1;**123**(4):364-373. DOI: 10.1161/CIRCULATIONAHA.110.971622

[116] Butler J, Hamo CE, Udelson JE, et al. Reassessing phase II heart failure clinical trials: Consensus recommendations. Circulation. Heart Failure. 2017 Apr;**10**(4):e003800. DOI: 10.1161/CIRCHEARTFAILURE.116.003800

[117] Halkos ME, Zhao ZQ, Kerendi F, et al. Intravenous infusion of mesenchymal stem cells enhances regional perfusion and improves ventricular function in a porcine model of myocardial infarction. Basic Research in Cardiology. 2008 Nov;**103**(6):525-536. DOI: 10.1007/s00395-008-0741-0

[118] Hamamoto H, Gorman JH 3rd, Ryan LP, et al. Allogeneic mesenchymal precursor cell therapy to limit remodeling after myocardial infarction: The effect of cell dosage. The Annals of Thoracic Surgery. 2009 Mar;**87**(3):794-801. DOI: 10.1016/j.athoracsur.2008.11.057

[119] Schuleri KH, Feigenbaum GS, Centola M, et al. Autologous mesenchymal stem cells produce reverse remodelling in chronic ischaemic cardiomyopathy. European Heart Journal. 2009 Nov;**30**(22):2722-2732. DOI: 10.1093/eurheartj/ehp265

[120] Hashemi SM, Ghods S, Kolodgie FD, et al. A placebo controlled, dose-ranging, safety study of allogenic mesenchymal stem cells injected by endomyocardial delivery after an

acute myocardial infarction. European Heart Journal. 2008 Jan;**29**(2):251-259. DOI: 10.1093/eurheartj/ehm559

[121] Teerlink JR, Metra M, Filippatos GS, et al. Benefit of cardiopoietic mesenchymal stem cell therapy on left ventricular remodelling: Results from the congestive heart failure Cardiopoietic regenerative therapy (CHART-1) study. European Journal of Heart Failure. 2017 May 31. DOI: 10.1002/ejhf.898

[122] Losordo DW, Henry TD, Davidson C, et al. Intramyocardial, autologous CD34+ cell therapy for refractory angina. Circulation Research. 2011 Aug 05;**109**(4):428-436. DOI: 10.1161/CIRCRESAHA.111.245993

[123] Perin EC, Borow KM, Silva GV, et al. A phase II dose-escalation study of allogeneic mesenchymal precursor cells in patients with ischemic or nonischemic heart failure. Circulation Research. 2015 Aug 28;**117**(6):576-584. DOI: 10.1161/CIRCRESAHA.115.306332

[124] Poglajen G, Sever M, Cukjati M, et al. Effects of transendocardial CD34+ cell transplantation in patients with ischemic cardiomyopathy. Circulation. Cardiovascular Interventions. 2014 Aug;**7**(4):552-559. DOI: 10.1161/CIRCINTERVENTIONS.114.001436

[125] Quyyumi AA, Waller EK, Murrow J, et al. CD34(+) cell infusion after ST elevation myocardial infarction is associated with improved perfusion and is dose dependent. American Heart Journal. 2011 Jan;**161**(1):98-105. DOI: 10.1016/j.ahj.2010.09.025

[126] Cui LL, Kinnunen T, Boltze J, et al. Clumping and viability of bone marrow derived mesenchymal stromal cells under different preparation procedures: A flow cytometry-based in vitro study. Stem Cells International. 2016;**2016**:1764938. DOI: 10.1155/2016/1764938

[127] Hemeda H, Giebel B, Wagner W. Evaluation of human platelet lysate versus fetal bovine serum for culture of mesenchymal stromal cells. Cytotherapy. 2014 Feb;**16**(2):170-180. DOI: 10.1016/j.jcyt.2013.11.004

[128] Astori G, Amati E, Bambi F, et al. Platelet lysate as a substitute for animal serum for the ex-vivo expansion of mesenchymal stem/stromal cells: Present and future. Stem Cell Research & Therapy. 2016 Jul 13;**7**(1):93. DOI: 10.1186/s13287-016-0352-x

[129] Amer MH, Rose FRAJ, Shakesheff KM, et al. Translational considerations in injectable cell-based therapeutics for neurological applications: Concepts, progress and challenges. npj Regenerative Medicine. 2017;**2**(1):23. DOI: 10.1038/s41536-017-0028-x

[130] Mamidi MK, Singh G, Husin JM, et al. Impact of passing mesenchymal stem cells through smaller bore size needles for subsequent use in patients for clinical or cosmetic indications. Journal of Translational Medicine. 2012 Nov 21;**10**(1):229. DOI: 10.1186/1479-5876-10-229

[131] Fernandez-Aviles F, Sanz-Ruiz R, Climent AM, et al. Global position paper on cardiovascular regenerative medicine. European Heart Journal. 2017 Sep 01;**38**(33):2532-2546. DOI: 10.1093/eurheartj/ehx248

[132] Knoepfler PS. Key action items for the stem cell field: Looking ahead to 2014. Stem Cells and Development. 2013 Dec;**22**(Suppl 1):10-12. DOI: 10.1089/scd.2013.0322

[133] Knoepfler PS. Call for fellowship programs in stem cell-based regenerative and cellular medicine: New stem cell training is essential for physicians. Regenerative Medicine. 2013 Mar;**8**(2):223-225. DOI: 10.2217/rme.13.1

[134] Martin PG, Martinez AR, Lara VG, et al. Regulatory considerations in production of a cell therapy medicinal product in Europe to clinical research. Clinical and Experimental Medicine. 2014 Feb;**14**(1):25-33. DOI: 10.1007/s10238-012-0213-6

[135] Schulman IH, Suncion V, Karantalis V, et al. Clinical research skills development program in cell-based regenerative medicine. Stem Cells Translational Medicine. 2015 Feb;**4** (2):118-122. DOI: 10.5966/sctm.2014-0144

[136] Goff ZD, Kichura AB, Chibnall JT, et al. A survey of unregulated direct-to-consumer treatment centers providing stem cells for patients with heart failure. JAMA Internal Medicine. 2017;**177**(9):1387-1388. DOI: 10.1001/jamainternmed.2017.2988

[137] Ancans J. Cell therapy medicinal product regulatory framework in Europe and its application for MSC-based therapy development. Frontiers in Immunology. 2012;**3**:253. DOI: 10.3389/fimmu.2012.00253

[138] Health USDo, Human Services F, Drug Administration CfBE, et al. Guidance for human somatic cell therapy and gene therapy. Human Gene Therapy. 2001 Feb 10;**12**(3):303-314. DOI: 10.1089/10430340150218431

[139] Sipp D, Caulfield T, Kaye J, et al. Marketing of unproven stem cell–based interventions: A call to action. Science Translational Medicine. 2017 Jul 05;**9**(397):eaag0426. DOI: 10.1126/scitranslmed.aag0426

[140] Chirba-Martin MA, Noble A. Our Bodies, our cells: FDA regulation of autologous adult stem cell therapies. Bill of Health. 2013

[141] Bianco P, Barker R, Brustle O, et al. Regulation of stem cell therapies under attack in Europe: For whom the bell tolls. The EMBO Journal. 2013 May 29;**32**(11):1489-1495. DOI: 10.1038/emboj.2013.114

[142] Cyranoski D. Stem cells in Texas: Cowboy culture. Nature. 2013 Feb 14;**494**(7436):166-168. DOI: 10.1038/494166a

[143] Preventive therapy. Nature. 2013 Feb 14;**494**(7436):147-148

[144] Smoke and mirrors. Nature. 2013 Apr 18;**496**(7445):269-270

[145] Yuan BZ, Wang J. The regulatory sciences for stem cell-based medicinal products. Frontiers of Medicine. 2014 Jun;**8**(2):190-200. DOI: 10.1007/s11684-014-0323-5

[146] Unknown territory. Nature. 2013 Feb 7;**494**(7435):5

[147] Simari RD, Moye LA, Skarlatos SI, et al. Development of a network to test strategies in cardiovascular cell delivery: The NHLBI-sponsored cardiovascular cell therapy research network (CCTRN). Journal of Cardiovascular Translational Research. 2010 Feb;**3**(1):30-36. DOI: 10.1007/s12265-009-9160-3

[148] Park KE, Moye LA, Henry TD, et al. Implementation of cardovascular cell therapy network trials: Challenges, innovation and lessons learned from experience in the CCTRN. Expert Review of Cardiovascular Therapy. 2013 Nov;**11**(11):1495-1502. DOI: 10.1586/14779072.2013.839943